The History
of the
Peanut Allergy
Epidemic

Heather Fraser

ISBN-10 1-449-91665-1

EAN-13 978-1-44991-665-7

Book cover design by David Whittaker, Useful Fictions

http://www.usefulfictions.co.uk

Peanut-designated tables in an elementary school lunchroom, Toronto, Ontario. Photo: Heather Fraser, 2009.
http://www.peanutallergyepidemic.com

Contents

Acknowledgements

As I read Margie Profet's "The Function of Allergy" (1991) I imagined an intensely curious woman who explored the odd angles of a question before finding something that finally made sense. Her example has been an inspiration.

Additional inspiration for this book has come from Generation Rescue, the autism community and the children and their parents who have taken a stand. Thank you for opening the door.

Children with food anaphylaxis and their families have occupied my thoughts for many years. I am grateful to them for their ongoing organized efforts to share information and to push forward laws that have helped protect vulnerable children. The most prominent example in this effort has been the Shannon family instrumental in the creation of Sabrina's Law.

How and why the epidemic of food allergy has occurred are enormous questions and I am grateful to everyone who has taken part in the discussion. To that end, my gratitude goes to the parents at the Canadian Vaccine Risk Awareness Network (VRAN) and the World Association of Vaccine Education (WAVE). I also am aware of the debt I owe to the many doctors who have conducted research and published their valuable findings on allergy and anaphylaxis.

My deep gratitude, as ever, goes to my friends David Whittaker and Ann Vink for their solid support as this project evolved. In addition, my special thanks go to Dr. Andrew Maniotis for his encouragement and Dr. Don Koval for his generous comments. I must also acknowledge my indebtedness to the community of holistic allergists in Canada and the US who have paved an excellent road to recovery from anaphylaxis. A special thank you to Susan Sethi for her courage and belief that recovery from anaphylaxis and autism can be achieved.

Many writers have provided me with material now woven into the spirit of this book. From the inquiries of the young Devi Lockwood to the stories of Deepak Chopra and Stephen Frye where neuropeptides met Greek tragedy during my long walks – I am grateful to them for stepping outside the box.

And finally, this book would have been impossible without Woody, Daisy and Rick. For my family unit, I am everlastingly grateful. To my family members John Fraser, Bill Tanner, Helen Boychuk as well as the extended clans, thank you for your encouragement. My mother, Sheila Horne deserves the lion's share of the credit for this book. She showed me the way.

Note to the Reader

Only puny secrets need protection. Big discoveries are
protected by public incredulity.

~ *Marshall McLuhan*

Information is instant, constant and exists all around us. This book is a product
of the era of information and communication: an individual can find an answer
to any question, if he is motivated.

I was motivated to write this book by an event for which I was completely
unprepared. In 1995, my first-born child at 13 months of age had an anaphylactic
reaction to peanut butter.

I wanted to know why.

The Problem of the Peanut Allergy

In 2009, the prevalence of peanut allergy in children living in the US, Britain, Canada and Australia was approximately 2% representing more than 2 million under 18 years of age.

In 1997 there were 416,400 peanut allergic American children,[1] a figure that more than doubled to 871,200 by 2002. In those 5 years, 454,800 children were sensitized to the food – an average of 90,960 each year before two years of age. And given that most children do not "outgrow" the allergy, there is today an increasing population of peanut allergic adults.

In 2009, 1.5% of the US population about 4.5 million people were peanut allergic.

Families with children allergic to peanuts (or any of the "Top 8" foods – tree nut, fish, shellfish, wheat, soy, dairy, egg[2]) live in a state of constant tension. If these families eat at restaurants, they do so with extreme caution. Not knowing the severity of the allergy, parents are vigilant for smears of peanut butter left on tables or on grocery cart handles. Trace amounts on the skin or lip or even the scent of the food could trigger a reaction. Parents, the child, caregivers and teachers are fearful. Children are segregated in school cafeterias at peanut tables, left out of play because friends have peanut butter in the house. Every school now tackles the peanut question, whether to ban peanut butter sandwiches and how to educate staff and students about the deadly nature of this ubiquitous childhood food.

Public awareness of peanut and other severe food allergies has impacted education systems and social norms, provoked legal reform and made billions of dollars for those active in the Food Allergy Industry. This industry's infrastructure consists of many overlapping allergy awareness groups, international allergy associations, medical researchers, pharmaceutical companies, allergy doctors, "free from" food makers and government regulators all of which support or are supported by the growing legions of food allergic children.

The inherent inertia of this industrious leviathan, however, has pushed the salient questions into the background: how has the peanut allergy epidemic developed and why is it continuing?

It is difficult to accept the startling increase in peanut allergy in just the last 20 years as coincidence or to chalk it up to genetic fluke. The challenge for any concerned medical professional has been to unearth the precise practical mechanism of sensitization common to these children – how did they become sensitized in the first place? And while there are a limited number of proven ways of "how to" make someone anaphylactic – ingestion, inhalation, through the skin, injection – no hypothesis of mass sensitization has yet connected any of these functional mechanisms to all the specific characteristics of the peanut allergy epidemic.

Researchers have considered skin creams that contain peanut oil, peanut consumption and parasite burden without satisfactorily explaining why just kids, why peanut, why such a sudden surge and why almost exclusively in western countries. Risk factors for developing the allergy have been explored but without conclusion. These include: maternal age, mode of delivery, levels of intestinal flora, heredity, even birth month and socio-economic status. Confusing matters further is a debate over the basic concept of allergy: is allergy the outcome of a roulette style genetic predisposition to immune dysfunction or is allergy an innate, purposeful immune response?

An important and clear distinction must be made between *sensitizing* someone to peanut and *launching* the allergic reaction. Sensitization is believed to occur when a protein bypasses the detoxifying process of the digestive system and becomes bonded with blood serum. This prompts specific blood cells to create antibodies that are then programmed to recognize the threatening protein – in this case peanut protein. The launching of an allergic reaction, on the other hand, occurs when the body is subsequently exposed to the protein and the antibodies trigger the biochemical players in the allergic reaction.

Lack of a standardized definition of anaphylaxis has hampered some studies where categories of "true" anaphylaxis mediated by Ig antibodies are compared with non-Ig anaphylaxis. This is less of a concern with peanut allergy where apparent consensus is that it is almost always Ig mediated.

Immunologloglobulins epsilon (called IgE) are sentries of the body. The job of the IgE is to patrol the fortress walls, mucous membranes, looking for peanut protein intruders. When they detect one of the many peanut protein epitopes (strings of amino acids that are numbered 1 through 8 and all called Ara h after *arachis hypogea*, Latin for peanut)[3] they alert the body which in turn lets loose the army, the body's immune system. A biochemical cascade is deployed which is damaging and potentially dangerous. It is typically characterized by coughing, shortness of breath, itchy skin hives, systemic leaking of blood vessels that causes swelling and potential asphyxia, vomiting, diarrhea. In severe reactions, blood pressure drops draining vital organs and causing the heart to stop.

Scientists have shown that the anaphylactic condition can be achieved by inhaling peanut protein if it is combined with a toxic additive. For example, doctors have created anaphylaxis in lab animals that inhaled a mixture of peanut and cholera.[4] The toxic bacteria functions as an "adjuvant", an additive that excites the immune system to form antibodies. It is suggested that the toxin and benign food can become in this way linked and both remembered by the immune system.[5] One wonders, then at the idea of an allergy to bacteria and the toxins produced by them. Allergy to bacterial toxins has been acknowledged for many years[6] [7] and can result in inflammation of the tonsils and adenoids[8] and even anaphylaxis.[9]

Researchers have not explored the role of adjuvants in peanut sensitization. They have preferred to focus only on the peanut proteins, their allergenicity and the ingestion of them as the most obvious elements in sensitization. They seemed to think that if they could pin point the initial exposure to these proteins, they could stop the epidemic. To this end, they have considered the ways in which peanuts are prepared (boiled vs. roasted), age when they are introduced to the child's diet, maternal diet and breast milk, even peanut oil used in nipple creams. Although it is possible to create the condition through simple ingestion, it is difficult. A healthy digestive system will neutralize any potentially sensitizing protein.

In fact, peanut consumption by mother or child may have no relevance in the epidemic proportions of this allergy. A 2006-07 study stated simply that it did not matter whether mothers ate peanuts or not, the same percentage of kids developed the allergy. Some children, whose mothers did not eat peanuts before, during or after pregnancy, still developed peanut allergy. Kids who had never been exposed to peanuts exhibited anaphylaxis on their first taste of it. Sweden, which has a low level of peanut consumption, has a higher prevalence of the allergy than the US. Israel, which has a high level of peanut consumption, has a low prevalence of the allergy.

Another puzzling feature of the epidemic is that the allergy appears with far less frequency or not at all in developing and largely non-westernized countries like

India, China and South Africa where consumption and use of peanuts is equal to or higher than it is in the west. It is suggested that Chinese children do not have the allergy because their peanuts are boiled. This is not a satisfactory explanation because, while boiling reduces peanut proteins, it does not eliminate them. And in other countries like India where the allergy is non-existent, peanuts are not always boiled but prepared in a variety of ways.

Ultimately, the idea of consumption is mired in conflicting information not the least of which is why the sudden appearance of the allergy in the west if both east and west have been consuming peanut in equal quantities for decades. Sensitization to peanut on such a massive scale, more researchers are coming to believe, is not by an oral route.

Today, thousands of research articles by doctors on the biology of the allergic reaction, clinical observations, and allergy management are available in prestigious periodicals. From this mound of information, doctors have developed and tend to favor two explanations for the current epidemic of peanut sensitized children. They are the Helminth Hypothesis and the Hygiene Hypothesis.

Helminths are worms that live in the human intestinal tract. It surprised researchers in the 1980s to discover that people heavily infected with worms had few allergies. One study confirmed that 90% of Venezuelan Indians living in the rainforest had worms but no allergies. 10% of rich Venezuelans living in the cities had light worm infections and 43% had allergies. In fact, helminths are so effective at suppressing allergies that some western doctors now offer "worm therapy" in which desperate allergy sufferers suppress their symptoms with a deliberate dose of eggs from the pig whipworm.[10]

From this "worms vs. wealth" observation researchers have developed an explanation for all allergies: because parasites and humans have co-evolved, they have a seeming symbiotic relationship in which parasites suppress allergic reactions while enjoying their human host. Without worms, the theory states, humans are unable to achieve homeostasis. In other words, immune dysfunction occurs due to lack of worms.

As an explanation for peanut allergy, the Helminth Hypothesis is inadequate. It cannot explain why primarily toddlers have become allergic or why to just the same limited list of foods, peanuts or any of the Top 8. And given that western countries have been largely unburdened by major helminth infections for decades, it does not explain the relatively recent accelerated increase of food allergy.

Another popular explanation for the rise in allergies grew from an observed correlation between the general decline in family size and the rise of allergy. It was proposed that unhygienic contact in large families – lots of siblings bringing illness home from school – was important for the development of a healthy immune system. The Hygiene Hypothesis suggests that overzealous cleaning, germ killing products, chlorinated water, antibiotics and vaccines have "protected" the west unnaturally. And as a result, the immune systems of first world children in particular, are sheltered from a natural microbial burden. Their immature immune systems are under-stimulated, dysregulated and, therefore, prone to random allergic sensitization. This malfunction is a product of an unburdened lifestyle.

The Hygiene Hypothesis is problematic in explaining peanut allergy. It does not consider the possibility that the immune systems of these children are not under-stimulated but rather over-stimulated by westernized approaches to toxic chemicals, drugs and vaccinations. In addition, the theory does not indicate a practical mechanism of mass sensitization that would explain the specificity of the Top 8 food allergens. Nor does it explain the sudden acceleration in food allergy.

These two favored explanations for the epidemic assume that allergy is a dysfunction, that the body has made a mistake in attacking a benign substance. And yet, the opposite may be true. Some suggest that allergy has an evolved purpose seen before the 20th century but provoked increasingly today by drugs and noxious pollutants in our air, water and food.

American researchers Rachel Carson (1907-1964), Theron G. Randolph (1906-1995) and evolutionary biologist Margie Profet (b. 1958) proposed that allergy is an evolved protective response. In 1991, Profet stated in "The Function of Allergy" that allergy is a final and often risky natural defense against toxins linked to benign substances. The IgE antibody is not, as it is generally characterized in medical literature, a rogue immune factor.[11] It is more akin to a hero provoked by toxins the body has deemed a deadly threat. The scratching, vomiting, diarrhea and sneezing are desperate attempts to eject a toxin as fast as possible. It is a risky reaction but one the body is programmed to unleash as a last ditch effort to protect itself. This event occurs when the general defenses have been insufficient in preventing a specific toxin from accessing the blood stream for a second time.

This is a provocative concept. However, because it was developed before the massive rise in peanut allergy it lacks specificity – again why just peanut and why so suddenly?

Conspicuous by its absence from current theories is the one mechanism that actually has a history of creating mass allergy - injection. Injection is examined in this book in some detail since it was the means by which the "founder" of anaphylaxis Dr. Charles Richet stumbled on "alimentary anaphylaxis" in humans and animals over 100 years ago. Richet concluded in 1913 that food anaphylaxis was a response to proteins that had evaded modification by the digestive system. Using a hypodermic needle, he was able to create the condition in a variety of animals – mammals and amphibians – proving that the reaction was not only universal but also predictable using the method of injection.

There are two lines of thought in the medical literature regarding injection as a mechanism of sensitization. The first is that injection, in the form of vaccination, merely "unmasks" genetic predispositions or tendencies to allergic "disease". In short, there is something wrong with the child and not the vaccine.

The second line of thought is that there is a causal relationship between vaccine ingredients and allergy – and although the "allergenicity" of vaccines is widely acknowledged, the literature carefully avoids the question of what kinds of allergies vaccines can create. One exception to this apparent rule is an admission by doctors that an outbreak of gelatin allergy in children starting in 1997 was indeed caused by a vaccine. In that year, gelatin made from boiled animals was included in the DPTa vaccine.

Quantities and qualities of adjuvant and other vaccine ingredients injected into westernized children changed dramatically between 1989 and 1994 in the US, UK, Canada, Australia and all World Health Organisation conforming countries. During those years, at least five new vaccine formulations for the same bacteria, Haemophilus influenzae type b (Hib) were introduced within an expanded and intense vaccination schedule. The fact that refined peanut oil is a common vaccine ingredient is a subject of concern equal to the potential of cross reactivity between the proteins of the Hib membrane and those in dietary peanut. Cross reactivity explains why a person who is allergic to peanut, a legume, may also react to nuts or citrus seeds[12] which belong to different plant families – their proteins have similar molecular weights.

As ingredients changed, the number of shots increased for kids in their first 18 months of life from 10 to as many as 29. The increase meant inconvenience to parents who would have to make more trips to the doctor and discomfort to the children, who would have to experience multiple injections. To overcome these obstacles to compliance with the new schedule, the vaccines for diphtheria, pertussis, tetanus (DPT), polio (OPV) and the Haemophilus influenzae b (Hib) were administered to children in a single visit with two injections and an oral polio dose starting in 1989. By 1994, these five were rolled into a single needle.

Paul Offit, Chief of Infectious Diseases at Children's Hospital in Philadelphia in 2008 dismissed concerns that the vaccination schedule was overwhelming children. To Offit, this was just not good science.[13] Other doctors disagreed. In respected medical journals such as *Journal of the American Medical Association* and *Allergy: European Journal of Allergy and Clinical Immunology* doctors expressed concern over the long-term effects of early vaccinations.[14] In Japan, childhood vaccination is delayed until two years of age. Some doctors go so far as to state that excessive vaccination is ineffective and dangerous.[15] [16]

But vaccination is a complex subject and its role in the allergy epidemic is difficult to address because of the heated political, social and economic implications. It is a subject doctors seem to avoid. And so, in spite of the continuing intense attention given to the peanut allergy epidemic, an answer has not yet been found. What has emerged instead is a robust economy of doctor fees, nut-free foods, medical research and pharmaceutical sales. Peanut and other food allergies have become enormously profitable. It is so much so that one market analyst has suggested that an "Autoimmune Index" would be a great tool for investors. This Index, tagged as "save the children and make money" would monitor the profitability of pharmaceutical stocks relative to the continued rise in peanut allergy and other childhood epidemics.[17]

Peanut allergy began as a mere idiosyncrasy after WW II. Today, its epidemic proportions help fuel a multi-billion dollar Food Allergy Industry.

Part 1

THE MYSTERY OF THE PEANUT ALLERGY EPIDEMIC

Chapter 1

From Idiosyncrasy to Multi-Billion Dollar Industry

Thirty-year-old Dr. Walter Teller disembarked from the Holland American liner Maasdam at New York City in December, 1954. Traveling from Germany, the young doctor had accepted a position at Mercy Hospital, Altoona, PA, and was greeted by his new colleagues at the pier. The men went to dinner in midtown. Five hours later, Dr. Teller was "nearly strangled" when his esophagus closed. He had eaten peanuts for the first time.

While a contemporary account of this event – possibly the first peanut reaction to be reported in the popular media – would reflect drama, fear and worry that a doctor could be so blithe about peanuts, at the time it was barely newsworthy. To the reporter who covered the story in five paragraphs, the allergic reaction was about as interesting as the doctor's car that, coincidentally, had been vandalized during that very dinner. Dr. Teller's unusual first evening in New York City was buried on page 31 in the Books section of the *New York Times*.[1][2]

Until the last decade of the 20th century, the US press typically met the rare and curious reactions to peanut with surprise and a shrug of the shoulders. It was just too hard to imagine that a common food could really be that dangerous even to the obvious victim. A rare feature on allergy in *Harper's Magazine* in 1939 delved into the defensive nature of these strange "food idiosyncrasies" that could cause swelling, sneezing, headaches, itching and rash but not death, it seemed.[3] In fact, allergy had a lighter side. A young woman's allergy helped her prove that a platinum necklace from her fickle sweetheart was actually nickel when she broke out in an allergic rash. And a restaurant patron proved by virtue of his swollen ankles that the economic waiter had merely scraped the anchovies off his eggs before re-serving them.

At this time, however, there was one exception to the anomalous nature of food allergies. Starting in the late 1930s there was a small but troubling outbreak of anaphylaxis to just one food, cottonseed oil. The outbreak startled doctors, government agencies and the food industry but, again, was not newsworthy. In the few reports about allergy at this time, cottonseed oil was mentioned as just one among many foods that caused reactions.[4]

In an investigation, however, the Food and Drug Administration (FDA) found that sloppy cottonseed crushing protocols had led to the contamination of many other oils subsequently used in processed foods. While this discovery explained how people were exposed unknowingly to the oil, it did not explain how so many had suddenly become sensitized to it. They had been consuming this oil for decades in the US without apparent problem. Doctors responded to the outbreak with a flurry of analyses and opinions none of which managed to unearth the functional cause of this mass sensitization.[5]

The rising prevalence of cottonseed allergy, however, resolved as quickly and as mysteriously as it had arrived.[6] Intense scrutiny in medical literature of this outbreak peaked during the late 1940s and sharply declined during the 1950s. This short-lived medical crisis was never fully investigated.

As reports of cottonseed allergy fell, peanut allergy emerged in US medical literature. Prevalence of this allergy, however, grew more slowly.

In 1941, well-known allergist Warren Vaughan, in his book *Strange Malady*, had dismissed peanut from his considerable list of potential food allergens. In his medical practice, Vaughan had seen allergies to milk, egg, corn, soybean, cottonseed, shrimp, tomato, cabbage, cherry, chocolate, strawberries and many more foods. Significantly, however, the doctor did not consider there to be any allergic concern about peanut. In fact, in the book he mentions crushed peanuts as a food topping without further comment.

And yet, by 1948, peanut sensitivity had become a serious "obstacle" in studies involving children and penicillin.[7]

Medical articles published in 1956, 1961 and 1963 reveal a growing interest in the increasingly common allergy to peanuts.[8] In fact, peanut and other severe food allergies soon affected so many people that with the peanut allergy death in 1972 of a 10-year-old Boston boy, Michael Grzybinski, there was a public outcry for proper food container labeling.

The media coverage of this tragedy revealed a far greater sympathy for food allergic people than had been exhibited in the 1950s over Dr. Teller's near death experience. The death of a child who ate "ice cream with peanut butter whipped into it" might have been prevented if the container had had its ingredients listed on the side, exclaimed a very upset Dr. Jean Mayer, Professor of Nutrition at Harvard University. The doctor wrote: "We think food manufacturers should no more be allowed to hide behind 'the need to protect recipe secrets' than drug manufacturers are. In both cases, lack of information can be not only unhealthy, but even deadly."[9]

The doctor's anger in albeit the limited press coverage is matched only by the sadness of the parents who in an open letter demanded that the FDA implement labeling laws. A deepening awareness of peanut as a deadly problem for a slim minority of children and adults found more room in newspapers from that moment on. Yet, the allergy was still not taken seriously. Throughout the 1970s, peanut allergy in the media was isolated to festive occasions like Christmas. Newspaper food section articles alerted the conscientious hostess to the potential of food allergy among her holiday guests. Peanut allergy was not a cause for widespread alarm.

And yet, doctors knew it was on the rise.

In 1973, the first formal US study of peanut allergy was launched by S.A. Bock who followed 114 children for 12 years concluding that none had outgrown his reactivity.[10] The report underlined the fact that children far more than adults developed food anaphylaxis and that peanut had emerged as a dangerous food that should be watched.[11] And so doctors watched the allergy, none publicly posing the obvious question – like the cottonseed oil mystery, what was causing people to become sensitized to this one food? An additional and surprising question this time, however, was why the allergy was rising almost exclusively in children.

But, rather than unearth the root cause of this mounting concern, doctors in 1980 chose instead to address the allergy after it had been established. In that year, medical researchers isolated the proteins that trigger the peanut reaction – Ara h 1 and 2. This was valuable information in the manufacture of vaccines and other allergy treatments. The growing problem of peanut and other food allergies was a market opportunity for pharmaceutical companies.

In 1980, the Epipen was introduced to allergists who prescribed them for patients. The EpiPen is a portable, emergency auto-injection of epinephrine. Epinephrine temporarily relaxes muscles and slows the allergic reaction. The EpiPen automatic syringe was licensed to Center Laboratories, NY from manufacturer Survival Technology, Inc. owned by physician Stanley J. Sarnoff. STI and inventor Shel Kaplan had patented the hypodermic injection device in

1977. The syringe was originally designed for the US military supplementing STI's other auto-injector that was used to administer a nerve gas antidote during battle.[12]

Commercial interests led the way in allergy management while social, legal and political initiatives lagged. Poor food labeling, again, was blamed for another death in 1980 of a 17-year-old boy. He had eaten a candy bar that contained peanuts.[13]

A turning point in media sympathy for peanut allergic children was marked by the death of an 18-year-old US national squash champion in 1986.[14]

This tragedy was followed by a new tone of sober inquiry into what the media perceived to be a serious and growing threat to children. A healthy and accomplished teenager had died after eating a spoonful of chili thickened with peanut butter. Headlines reflected new vigor in bringing information to the public including population studies and a review of emergency measures.

The media challenged restaurants to list ingredients and airlines to consider in-flight peanut restrictions.[15] Of new import as well for the first time was interest in an explanation for this child-specific allergy – thoughts turned naturally to mothers' diets while pregnant and breastfeeding. In 1941, allergist Warren Vaughan had already fingered the "abnormal food cravings"[16] of pregnant women as the source of allergens to which children often become sensitized. But this educated guesswork did not explain the rising prevalence of allergy to peanut when this dietary staple had been consumed for decades without obvious problem. One reporter looked fearfully to an allergy filled future following the 1987 death of an 11 year old asthmatic boy who had eaten peanut contaminated cake: "Every week brings reports of new dangers, a death from allergy…"[17]

Refreshed marketing efforts for EpiPens in 1988 introduced the word anaphylaxis to the mainstream media. News reports for the life-saving emergency device exploited the story of the 1986 death from peanut butter "laced" chili. An EpiPen might have saved her life. An article to this effect ran in the newspapers of six US cities in the summer of 1988.[18]

Starting around 1990, while the media continued to buzz about EpiPens, new allergy guides, cookbooks, labeling concerns, holiday season dangers, the biology of "when your immune system panics",[19] that it can be passed via organ transplant, and even whether the allergy was an over-diagnosed malady,[20] the prevalence of peanut allergy in children suddenly accelerated. Unnoticed by the public, hospital emergency room (ER) records in Australia, the UK and the US documented the upward momentum of food anaphylaxis admissions for children under five.

In the US, ER records showed a steady and rapid increase in anaphylaxis discharges between 1992 and 1994 from 467 per 100,000 to 671. This number jumped to 876 in 1995. In three years from 1992-95 the numbers nearly doubled. A 1991 US study determined that 90% of all food allergy fatalities were due to ingestion of peanut/tree nuts.[21] [22]

In the Australia Capital Territory (ACT), a four-fold increase in hospital admission rates for food allergy was observed from 1993 through 2004-5. ACT is a self-governing state within New South Wales with the highest density population and smallest area at 2,358 km². Within it is the national capital of Canberra. A 12-year study of allergy services in ACT showed a 400% increase for this period for children under five. During the course of the study, birth rates actually fell 10%. One allergist in Australia referred to this trend in allergy in children as an "epidemic".[23]

In hindsight, what was called the "the tip of the iceberg"[24] by University of Edinburgh allergist Aziz Sheikh in a 2006 lecture, the discharge rates for system allergic disorder in England increased between 1990 and 2001 from 1,960 admissions for allergic conditions to 6,752. This seven-fold jump in just 11 years indicated "a highly significant increase" in admissions for severe allergy.

The timing of this acceleration was confirmed by a UK peanut allergy study. A retrospective cohort analysis of children born between Jan. 1989 and Feb. 1990 on the isolated Isle of Wight, revealed a shocking statistic: by ages four and five in 1994, .5% of these children were anaphylactic to peanut and 1.1% showed sensitivity.[25] [26]

This news made riveting headlines. Not only were 40,000 UK children under four years of age "in peril from peanuts" but also they could react as one child did, to just its vapor.[27]

A second cohort analysis from the Isle of Wight provided an even bigger shock. An analysis of children born in the same region between Sept. 1, 1994 and Aug. 31, 1996 and tested at ages three and four, revealed that twice as many children were now allergic to peanuts: 1.1% were anaphylactic and 3.3% were sensitized.[28] [29] Again, the UK headlines ran sensational stories such as, "One bite and he dies" and "Rise of the killer food".[30]

Allergy to peanut in UK preschoolers had more than doubled in just four years and no one knew why.

Two other startling facts emerged around this time. The first was that 9% of Americans had "serologic evidence" of sensitivity to peanuts according to the US Centre for Disease Control's National Health and Nutrition Examination Survey (NHANE III data was collected from 1988 to 1994).[31] In other words, about 22 million people in the US had somehow become sensitized to peanut even if they were not actively reacting.

The second fact was that peanut allergy appeared to be a concern only in western countries. In China, for example, where peanut consumption was as high as in the west, the allergy was virtually unknown. Researchers suggested that the difference lay in the way peanuts were prepared. The Chinese often boiled their peanuts[32] that reduced their allergenicity while Americans roasted their peanuts, a process which intensified it. This explanation had many problems not the least of which was that if both countries had been eating peanuts for decades without seeming problem, why the sudden prevalence and why just in children. As well, the mode of preparation theory did not hold true for India where peanut was prepared in a variety of ways, including roasting, and the allergy was also not known to exist.

While the mystery deepened, doctors continued to focus on post-sensitization treatments such as vaccination and allergy "shots". Both treatments were fraught with problems given the potential severity of the allergy.[33] A 1991 desensitizing experiment in Denver was nearly derailed by an accidental death. While it was reported that three patients in the study experienced diminished reactions to peanut after their shots, a 15-year-old boy died when he received an incorrect injection dosage.[34] A pharmacist received two years probation for this death. Looking back from 2006, allergist Hugh Sampson was quoted as saying that in this and other such trials "everybody was getting significant adverse reactions throughout. So it was decided that standard immunotherapy was not a reasonable way to go."[35]

The "Ultimate allergy shot," was made public in Jan. 1995 by Peptide Therapeutics in the UK.[36] It was potentially "one of the biggest selling drugs ever". The company had already raised £4.5 Million and was ready for human clinical trials. A news report explained that the vaccine worked by provoking the body to generate IgG antibodies that suppress IgE, the "allergy antibodies". The UK vaccine, however, appeared to fall from the spotlight as quickly as it had emerged.

In the US, research and clinical trials using a vaccine TNX-901 to reduce sensitivity to peanut were ultimately axed during a much-publicized squabble over rights between two pharmaceutical giants.[37]

Meanwhile, EpiPen sales were growing. In 1992, Centre Labs in New York paired with Fisons Pharmaceuticals to distribute marketing material that claimed 15% of the US population, 3.8 million people had life threatening allergies to drugs and foods[38] all of whom would be reached by their team of 350 sales reps visiting primary care physicians and pediatricians across the US. Their smaller sales team of 15 would continue to sell to allergy doctors. EpiPen ads appeared in medical journals like the *Journal of the American Medical Association* (JAMA). Retailing at $30. in 1992, about 400,000 EpiPens were sold in the US and the marketers hoped to sell one million more over the next two years for gross sales of $15 Million.[39] The US retail price of an EpiPen was between $64. and $118. in 2009.

A real comprehension of the danger posed by peanut to a minority of children dawned more slowly on public school staff members. In 1994, a frightened mother learned that a lunchroom aide at her son's elementary school had forced her six-year-old peanut allergic son to bite a nut cookie.[40] The private UN International School in New York made headlines when a peanut allergic five year old was denied entry after his mother refused to sign a waiver of responsibility.[41] One creative allergist and a Mom of an allergic two year old thought allergy badges might help at schools and daycares. Shirts emblazoned with badges of bright yellow, green and pink would single out the fatally allergic.[42]

This double-edged idea did not catch on. Doctors had warned of psychological issues related to wearing Epipen belts and badges would be no less problematic.

Peanut allergy tipped into critical mass in the early-1990s when a "sudden surge of severely allergic children entering school systems…caught many educators off guard."[43] A teacher writing in 2000 recalled the surprising phenomenon of the flood of four and five year old food allergic children. Schools were obliged by law to deal with the enormous social, medical and logistical problems of protecting handfuls of peanut and other food allergic kindergarten children in each school. There were thousands of these children across school boards and soon there were millions across the US, Canada and other western countries. This eyewitness to the surge confirmed by ER records plus the Isle of Wight cohort studies pointed to these few years – the late 1980s and early 90s – as the starting point of the accelerated prevalence of peanut allergy in children.

Society was unaware that anything had happened until the affected children showed up for kindergarten.

By 1996, some schools had created peanut free zones while others attempted to ban peanuts altogether as they did in Massachusetts.[44] One school in North Andover that banned peanuts had five kindergarten students with peanut allergy. These kids were assigned to the same peanut free class, all substances including the hand soap were checked for hidden ingredients, and all parents were told to leave the peanut butter at home. And yet, some felt the peanut ban was not the best solution. "Peanut bans don't work," stated Ms. Munoz-Furlong in 1996, founder of the Food Allergy and Anaphylaxis Network (FAAN).[45] A peanut free status suggested to people that they were safe "and that's dangerous. They let their guard down."

Most schools, however, did not have policies or procedures and certainly there were no laws. In this unprotected vacuum, parents grew fearful and refused to let their allergic kids attend field trips envisioning their reactive child trapped on a bus with the food. These parents strapped Epi-belts on the children, and taught them how to use the auto-injector not yet trusting schools to have this medication at the ready. They profiled their allergic children in laminated homemade posters placed strategically in schools.

Most kindergarten children ate their lunches in their classroom, so initially only individual classrooms were made peanut free. As more allergic children entered school behind the initial group, they were accommodated in lunchrooms with separate tables. In some schools, the section was signed "Peanut Tables" with

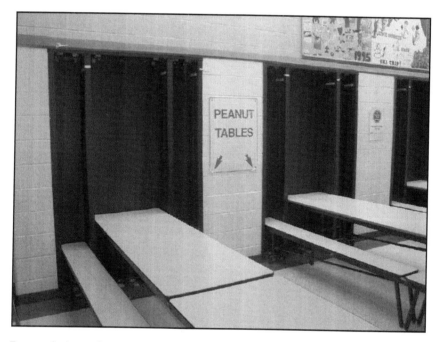

Peanut-designated tables in an elementary school lunchroom, Toronto, Ontario.

red arrows segregating the expanding number of allergic children. Lunch bag inspections became common. Any peanut related food, granola bar or sandwich, was confiscated and sent home with a cautionary note.

Parents of peanut allergic children incurred the enmity of the, as yet, not understanding parents of the non-allergic children. This latter group of parents insisted that the peanut butter ban had violated their rights. "A staple was under fire," screamed a 1996 headline.[46] Peanut butter, a cheap and tasty source of protein, had been a staple of lunch boxes for decades. Eventually, more and more schools went peanut free with varying degrees of success given the enormity of the task.

In 1998, behavior related peanut, nuts and allergic children noticeably impacted family grocery buying habits – the growth of the "free from" food market category was a concrete index of the epidemic having hit critical mass. That year the Swiss based food giant Nestle, responded to this market reality with a line of chocolate bars made in a "peanut free facility". Targeting concerned adults, Nestle marketed their "peanut free promise" with Halloween food safety.

Halloween generates the greatest sales volume of sweets for the entire year. According to a Nielsen market report, chocolate sales in 2008 accounted for $1.2 Billion of the total $1.9 Billion of candy sales. In 2001, 41 million trick-or-treaters filled their bags with candy. Other savvy food manufacturers soon jumped on board with allergen free products for children (cookies, candy, ice cream) and cautious labeling.

The peanut segment of the snack market fell from 14.4% to 12.4% between 1993 and 1999. The shrinking supply-managed peanut industry[47] remained sluggish in large part due to the growth in peanut allergy concerns.[48] The important youth market segment of children under 14 was in decline. In 2008, it was recommended that peanut industry leaders not wait for the health care industry to fix the allergy problem and to take matters into their own hands by producing a transgenic, allergen-free peanut.

In 2003, biotech giant Monsanto began to grow genetically engineered peanuts in India. By 2007,[49] these peanuts were approved for growth in the US by the American Peanut Council. Urging due diligence on the part of scientists, the Council claimed that an engineered peanut could be safer, more nutritious and easier to grow than conventional versions. At Georgia University, Peggy Ozias-Akins, a professor of plant biology, began researching how to erase "allergen" genes in peanut plants as well as adding separate genes for disease resistance.

Legal systems were also challenged by the peanut allergy epidemic. In 2000, the family of an Australian woman received a multi-million dollar settlement from a restaurant after it had served her peanut contaminated food. Her anaphylactic reaction had caused brain damage.[50]

In 2006, the Ontario provincial government passed Sabrina's Law, a non-punitive expectation that all schools would comply with training, practices and education in life threatening allergies.[51] By 2008, the Ontario public school system had over 40,000 anaphylactic students whose biographies with allergy profiles and photos decorated the walls of every teachers lounge ensuring that the entire community was aware of their status. Today most, if not all, westernized countries have adopted policies on food allergy and its management in schools and childcare centres. In 1999, the US courts confirmed that under the Americans with Disabilities Act schools and day care centers must accommodate an individual's peanut allergy.[52] In 2006, the US government introduced the Food Allergy and Anaphylaxis Management Act providing public K to 12 schools with voluntary emergency guidelines.

While most people in the school community showed due concern for allergic kids, the "allergy bully" did not. Charges were laid in a groundbreaking 2008 felony case when a Kentucky 8th grader was accused of placing peanut butter cookie crumbs in the lunch box of another student.[53] And again in 2008, jail time was given to a 19-year-old Wenatchee Washington student who smeared peanut butter on the face of an allergic classmate.[54]

In spite of the evidence, doctors still seemed polarized on the magnitude of peanut allergy problem. One doctor who pointed out that more people die from lightning strikes than from peanut, called the peanut paranoia a mass psychogenic illness.[55] He referred to current behavior of parents and school staff as epidemic hysteria citing the evacuation of a school bus full of 10 year olds after a single peanut was spotted on the floor.[56] Yet another doctor, exasperated British Member of Parliament, Baroness Finlay of Llandaff called for increased funding for research and special allergy centres.[57] She was "extremely alarmed" about Department of Health guidance given to pregnant mothers telling them to avoid peanuts.

At the end of the day, the questions "how and why is this happening?" remained unanswered. What emerged instead in response to the mystery was a massive Food Allergy Industry the infrastructure of which included billions of dollars in the sale of free-from foods, web sites, blogs, magazines, parent initiated lobby groups such as Food Allergy Initiative (est. 1998, faiusa.org) or the Anaphylaxis Campaign (est. 1994 in the UK), doctor initiated associations such as Food and Allergy Anaphylaxis Network (est. 1991, http://www.foodallergy.org/) and the many allergy and immunology associations for doctors and umbrella associations in western countries such as the World Allergy Organization.

There was much overlap between the organizations and all either created their own conferences or took part in annual trade shows that were in turn supported by fundraisers, private donations, government grants and pharmaceutical companies.[58] Pharmaceuticals – allergy drugs, testing and medical research – made up an enormous part of the billions spent each year. During 2004, 1,511,534 EpiPen prescriptions were filled in the US representing 2,495,188 EpiPens.[59] Registries such as Allergovigilance Network in France, the Food Allergy Register in Norway or the ILSI European Food Allergy Task Force in Belgium began to collect data on anaphylactic reactions. Europrevall, a €14M project brought together over 53 research centres to investigate food allergy.

The WHO's Codex Alimentarius provided a handy Top 8 list of "critical food allergens" – peanuts, tree nuts, dairy, egg, wheat, crustacean, fish, soybeans – and a downgraded list of 160 foods reported as able to provoke severe reactions. These lists and concomitant guidelines on their use in the food industry was a doubled edged sword – useful on the one hand but invasive in the sense that the World Trade Organization (WTO) upheld WHO Codex Alimentarius guidelines in all trade disputes. This encouraged legislative change that forced manufacturers in many countries to comply with "guidelines". With the increasing reliance on and power given to WHO guidelines, it was proving problematic that the WHO had deemed it unnecessary to list, for example, refined peanut oil on food labels. This guideline extended to pharmaceutical labeling due to its GRAS status (generally recognized as safe) in the US. Many pharmaceutical products including vitamins and vaccines historically have contained refined peanut oil and continued to include it without informing the consumer. Corporate law also shielded exact ingredients of patented pharmaceuticals.

With such intense activity and the proliferation of so much money it was easy to lose sight of the presumed goal – unearthing the functional mechanism of sensitization – what was causing children to become sensitized to peanut in the first place?

To that end, doctors examined with mixed and often conflicting results, the risk factors for developing peanut allergy.

Chapter 2

Risk Factors

In successive waves through the 1990s, hundreds of thousands of peanut allergic children arrived for kindergarten at public schools across the US, Canada, Australia, the UK and many other western countries. Critical mass, it seemed, was achieved almost overnight catching educators off guard and prompting sudden changes in social behavior, shopping and eating habits. Doctors had watched for years as prevalence of the allergy slowly climbed. With this unanticipated acceleration, a sense of urgency and desperation marked the medical literature. Researchers analyzed any feature no matter how unlikely that seemed to distinguish peanut allergic children from others.

The only thing that seemed clear was that the most commonly held risk factors such as eating peanuts had little or no apparent relevance in the epidemic proportions of the allergy. Risk factors like atopy, maternal age, cesarean birth, socio-economic status and heredity were seen to contribute to allergic tendency but none explained the specificity of the peanut or its sudden prevalence. Even geography was a misleading factor since it had been used as a convenient way to demarcate patterns of food consumption.[1] For this allergy, neither consumption of peanuts nor methods of their preparation or cultivation were relevant. Geography did hold significance but for a new pattern of toxicity seemingly specific to the western lifestyle. A profile of the person most liable to develop a peanut allergy emerged from the known risk factors: a toddler (male 2:1) born after 1990 whose ability to detoxify was somehow impaired.

Geography

Geography was believed to be a primary risk factor for developing the allergy. An acknowledged but puzzling feature of the allergy was that it seemed to exist only in western countries – the UK, parts of Europe, Canada, the US and Australia. Doctors were quite convinced that it simply did not exist in developing and eastern countries such as China, India or parts of Africa. In fact, explanations for the general rise in allergies such as the Hygiene Hypothesis rested on this east vs. west observation. Starting in 2005, however, reports of peanut allergy in unexpected prevalence emerged from Hong Kong, Ghana and Singapore. When word of these new outbreaks reached the medical community, the response was utter silence. No one could explain it.

The first reports regarding these new outbreaks indicated only serologic evidence with limited actual reactivity, but that quickly changed. By 2008, severe peanut reactions in children living in Hong Kong had increased: 1% of children aged two to seven were found to be allergic.

And in Cape Town, South Africa, again serologic evidence of peanut sensitivity was found in 5% of children studied although reactivity was limited and non-anaphylactic. The reason for this hypo-reactivity was already well known. Helminths or intestinal worms dampened every immune reaction and these children were heavily infested.

But doctors had failed to notice a trend in the way the allergy suddenly emerged. A similar phenomenon had occurred in the US. In 1994, 9% of US population was reported to be sensitized to peanut although the vast majority was non-reactive. By 1997, .6% of American children were reactive but, as in Hong Kong, this number quickly rose.

Taking this observation to a logical extreme, if sensitization grew at the same rate as documented reactivity in children, by 2003 13% of the US population – 38,220,000 million people – would be sensitized to peanut. In 2003, an estimated 1.04% of the US population was reactive to peanuts. Were the numbers then about 1:13: three million actively peanut allergic people for every 38 million sensitized? If that was true, whole populations were rapidly being sensitized to their own food.

Using that modest percentage of 1.04% in 2003[2] for the top five countries, the total peanut allergic population for 2003 was more than 4.3 million people: 3,057,600 in the US; 327,704 in Canada; 613,600 in the UK; 92,332 in Sweden; 205,165 in Australia. Although difficult to confirm, some believe this number in 2009 to have risen to an estimated 2% of these populations – 7.36 million people.

Tracking the growth of peanut allergy from the start was a little like train spotting. Data was generated in small, isolated studies that was then shared obsessively across the Internet and in medical journals. The upward trend continued to be monitored in the UK and Australia, in particular. And yet in other countries – Norway, Denmark and Germany and Japan – prevalence of the allergy was low (see Appendix). In Estonia, Lithuania and Russia, the allergy was of limited or no significance. And in the Sub-Sarhara and India, it was virtually non-existent. The numbers of peanut allergic children included[3]:

- 1.71+% (2007) Canadian children
- 1.2+ % (2002) US children
- 2+% (2009) UK children
- .45+% (2002) French children
- 1.2+% (1998) Swedish children
- .5% (2005) Danish children
- .17% (2006) Israeli children

- .53% (2009) Ghana, African children
- 1.11% (2009) Australian children living in Tasmania
- 2% (2009) Australian children living in the Australian Capital Territory
- 1.08%-1.35% (2008) Singaporean children
- .57% - 1% (2009) Chinese children living in Hong Kong

Peanut consumption

Ingestion of peanuts was believed to be another primary risk factor for developing the allergy. Researchers looked closely at methods by which peanuts were prepared, where they were grown, levels and modes of exposure to them before and after birth. They were surprised to learn, ultimately, that just eating peanuts had no relevance in the epidemic proportions of the allergy.

Boiling peanuts was thought to be the reason for the virtual non-existence of the allergy in children living in China. This method of preparing peanuts reduced their allergenic proteins. Roasting on the other hand, a common method of preparation in the US, tended to enhance their allergenicity. However, using this observation to explain the lack of prevalence of the allergy in China proved difficult. Intact peanut proteins were still being consumed. As well, the allergy was not known to exist in India where peanuts were prepared in a variety ways, including roasted. And finally, the emergence of the allergy in Hong Kong and Singapore, where boiling peanuts was ostensibly the preferred method of preparation, completely upended the idea.

And farming methods and differences in soil were found to have no bearing on allergenicity of the peanut. Whether grown in Israel, India or Kentucky, peanut proteins were the same.[4]   Note has been made of the fact that peanuts also contain histamine and other substances that may affect allergenicity. No research has yet been conducted on these in relation to proteins.[5]

Level of consumption appeared to have no bearing on the epidemic either. In Sweden, where consumption of peanut was low, prevalence of the allergy in children was the same as it was in the US.[6] The inverse was true for Israel where consumption was high and prevalence was low.

And so, perplexed researchers turned next to analyze the allergic child and the tender age at which he first consumed peanut.

The most debated risk factor related to peanut consumption was whether or not consumption by pregnant and nursing mothers contributed to the prevalence of the allergy. Through the late 1990s medical opinion on the issue swung from one extreme to the other – should mothers eat peanuts or stay away from them – without consensus.

Some believed sensitization occurred in utero, before the child was born.[7] Others suggested it occurred during breastfeeding or through ingestion of refined peanut oil in baby formula. Some considered that since IgE antibodies do not cross the placenta, perhaps peanut proteins did and that perhaps fetuses swallowed IgE from amniotic fluid that then resulted in sensitization.[8] Doctors believed they had evidence from aborted fetal tissues showing that from the second trimester onwards fetuses were capable of producing an allergic reaction. In a French study of 54 infants who were less than 11 days of age and 71 who were 17 days to four months of age, 8% had a positive skin prick test for peanuts.[9]

Another doctor urged that there was a lack of convincing evidence that manipulation of maternal diet during pregnancy had lasting effect on development of food allergy. And therefore, it was thought lactation was a more likely route of primary sensitization.[10] Yet, another study found no association at all between allergy and maternal peanut consumption while pregnant and breastfeeding.[11]

A provocative university dissertation in 2007 determined that avoidance of peanut reduced the prevalence of the allergy but only in the child's first year of life.[12] Avoidance had no benefit after age one. The author admitted that this was difficult to explain. She suggested that there could be a "subtle" and as yet undiscovered environmental exposure to sensitizing proteins.

Ultimately, a worried British Dept. of Health issued a warning to pregnant and nursing mothers who had a history of atopy (other allergies) to avoid peanuts and all nuts to prevent peanut allergy. In 1998, the UK Committee on Toxicity of Chemicals in Food, Consumer Products and the Environment issued a statement of avoidance.[13] The American Academy of Pediatrics also recommended delayed introduction of peanuts until three years of age for infants with a family history of allergies and maternal avoidance of peanuts during pregnancy and breastfeeding for mothers of such infants.[14] Observation that exposure to peanut oil hidden in vitamin supplements, nipple ointments, or soy formulae may contribute to sensitization was not rigorously examined. However, doctors had found some children were sensitized in this manner and some even reacted.[15 16 17]

And yet, not only did this avoidance strategy have no effect on reducing prevalence of the allergy but also it resulted in the highest number of peanut allergic children yet seen in the UK.[18] One study put the number at 2.8% of children. A report to the UK parliament in 2007 concluded simply that this seemingly sensible government advice may have made things worse.[19]

And so, doctors made a complete about face and asked whether it would be better for pregnant and nursing mothers to embrace peanuts and eat significant quantities of them. Exposure to peanuts during childhood was now thought to be crucial in developing immunological tolerance – it might even prevent the allergy. Conversely, a lack of peanuts could enhance sensitization.

A study in which English and Israeli children were compared concluded that the early introduction of peanuts in an Israeli baby food called "bamba" may have promoted tolerance and prevented peanut allergy.[20] In two populations of Jewish children ages four to 18 in Tel Aviv and London, researchers looked at the roles of timing, frequency and quantity of peanut consumption in the development of the allergy. The prevalence of the allergy was 1.85% in London and .17% in Israel. Among children ages four through 12, the prevalence was 2.05% in England and .12% in Israel. When analysis was restricted to those at high risk for peanut allergy, those with confirmed eczema, the prevalence was 6.46% in England and .79% in Israel. By nine months of age, 69% of Israeli infants and 10% of English infants were eating peanuts. The main source was peanut butter made from roasted peanuts.

But if reduced exposure to peanut proteins led to allergy, then the protein reduced boiled peanuts consumed in China should actually have created scores of peanut allergic kids. The early introduction theory made little sense especially in consideration of the prevalence of sesame allergy in Israel. Sesame allergy in Israel was almost as high as peanut allergy was in the UK. Ironically, Israeli studies claimed that the prevalence of this allergy in children was the result of their exposure to it too early in life.[21]

Ultimately, the LEAP study (The Learning Early About Peanut Allergy study scheduled for completion in 2013) emerged as a way to settle the issue of when and how to consume peanuts, to determine what was the best dietary strategy for prevention of the allergy.[22] Enrolled in the study were 640 children, 11 months or younger diagnosed with eczema or egg allergy or both. The LEAP study was sponsored by the US National Institutes of Health and coordinated by the Immune Tolerance Network, with support from the Food Allergy Initiative.

In an odd twist, lead researcher on this team suggested that eating peanuts may have a limited role to play in sensitization: "The index allergic reaction usually occurs soon after the first known oral ingestion – which suggests that peanut sensitization does not always occur via the oral route."[23] Some doctors simply admitted that the exact route of primary sensitization was unknown although the gastrointestinal (GI) immune system was likely to play an important role.[24]

The GI system was long understood to play a significant role in allergies. For one, the successful catalytic effects of enzymes on proteins is crucial to limiting the movement of complete proteins into the blood stream through the compromised and permeable tissue of the bowel wall. In this way, proteins are allowed to bind with blood serum resulting sensitization and allergic symptoms on exposure. Consuming the same food daily would increase the chances of developing an allergy to it.

Allergist Ken Bock suggested that low-grade infection in the GI tract would encourage allergic sensitization. Inflammation from such an infection sends out immune cell messengers that trigger even more inflammation in distant parts of the body. It can result in inflammation in joints, the lining of the GI tract and even the brain. All inflammation, Bock suggested, contributes to allergies.[25]

But as for simple consumption, in 2007 a report from the UK House of Lords Science and Technology committee confessed that levels of consumption by mothers or children appeared to have no relevance in the increasing prevalence of the allergy.[26] They offered that consumption of peanuts was up to individual discretion in consultation with a doctor.

The act of eating peanuts as a mechanism for mass sensitization was at the least mired in conflicting information. At the worst, it was like seeing a tree but missing the forest. While it was possible to develop anaphylaxis from just eating peanut, it would not cause an epidemic of anaphylaxis in millions of children, just in western countries, and with such abrupt prevalence. The epidemic proportions of peanut sensitized and anaphylactic children in this light appeared not to be directly connected with ingestion of the food whether early or late in childhood, whether boiled, roasted or served up in breast milk.

Atopy

Atopy from the Greek "atopos" which means "out of place" is a medical term used to describe a tendency of an individual toward allergic conditions like eczema and asthma. Atopy that indicates increased levels of IgE antibodies is a generally accepted risk factor in the development of additional allergies.[27] Doctors were divided, however, on its relevance in the peanut allergy epidemic.

In a cohort study of American children referred for the evaluation of atopic dermatitis between 1990 and 1994 the prevalence of allergic reactivity to peanuts was nearly twice as high as that in a similar group evaluated between 1980 and 1984.[28] A 1996 study concluded that peanut allergy was rarely an isolated manifestation of atopy.[29] A Melbourne study of 620 atopic Australian infants in 1997 indicated that 1.9% were peanut allergic although egg (2%) and milk (3.2%) were more common at age two.[30]

In contrast, according to a 2006 study of children in Israel and the UK, the propensity to atopy did not explain the increasing prevalence of peanut allergy. Atopy was as prevalent in the UK children as those in Israeli while peanut allergy was very low in Israel and high in the UK. Despite the study's unsteady conclusion that prevalence was related to a lack of early exposure (see "Peanut Consumption" above) it suggested that peanut allergy was independent of atopy. The allergy was seen in both supposed low risk and high-risk children. The differences in peanut allergy could not, in this study, be explained by generalized differences in atopy.[31]   The LEAP web site found that just 20% of children with atopy (especially eczema or egg allergy) also developed peanut allergy.

But what was causing the atopy?   Was atopy genetic and independent of peanut allergy or was there perhaps another underlying element that coincidentally linked both allergic conditions in children?

In 1997, one group of researchers thought they had found the connection. A Christchurch, New Zealand, longitudinal study followed 1,265 children born in 1977, 23 of which did not receive DPT and polio vaccinations. The non-vaccinated children had no recorded asthma episodes or consultation for asthma or other allergic illness before 10 years of age. In the immunized children, 23.1% had asthma episodes, 22.5% asthma consultations, and 30% had consultations for other allergic illnesses. Similar differences were observed at ages five and 16 years.

This study pointed to the pertussis toxin as having a direct IgE inducing effect. Two other factors that promoted atopy in children were the aluminum based vaccine adjuvants and the reduction in clinical infections in infancy.[32]

In the process of building healthy immunity, the period from birth to six months of age was considered to be crucial. Some believed that certain vaccines had altered this process leading to atopy.[33] [34]

At the same time, however, Japanese researchers saw an inverse association between tuberculin responses and atopic disorder: exposure and response to M. tuberculosis in a BCG vaccination appeared to inhibit atopic disorder through the lowering of serum IgE.[35]   10 years later, researchers found the opposite stating that there was an absence of relationships between tuberculin responses and adult atopy[36] and that the data was inconclusive.[37]

Doctors danced uncomfortably around the relationship of allergy and vaccination through the 1990s until finally the discussion was sidelined by a new and all encompassing concept of allergy and immunity – the Th1-Th2 paradigm. This model of immune function argued that a balanced immune system could be disrupted by any number of factors, not just vaccination. Poor nutrition, vitamin supplements, parasite infection, lack of parasite infection, disease or lack of disease could lead to atopy. The role of vaccination in atopy and allergy was thus engulfed by a massive construct that reduced it to just one of many immune altering exposures.

TH1 – TH2 Paradigm dysregulation

Doctors religiously have cited a general malfunction of the immune system as a risk factor for peanut allergy in children. The "Th1-Th2 paradigm" neatly organized the immune system by splitting it into two sides with two distinct T (thymus) white blood cell responses to pathogens and allergens. Doctors suggested that an upset in the balance between the two sides would almost certainly result in allergies. While it was a handy concept, the paradigm was later stickered as so much dogma unlikely to explain something as highly complex as the immune system. And as a risk factor in the epidemic, a dysregulation of the Th1-Th2 paradigm was not linked specifically to peanut allergy. It was just too broad.

White blood cells called T cells (matured in the thymus) and B cells (matured in bone marrow) circulate in the lymph, spleen, skin and gastro intestinal tract where they react with antigens (ie. bacteria, viruses). B cells proliferate and produce quantities of different antibodies including IgE (Immunoglobulin epsilon) the antibody most associated with atopy and allergy to deal with invaders that are outside the cells of the body (ie. allergens). The B cells rely in part on information from T cells.

T cells deal with invaders that cause damage inside cells (ie. viruses). They secrete cytokines (cell movers). There are two categories of T cells: cytotoxic T cells (killer T cells) that kill infected cells; and helper T cells which enhance responses of other cells like macrophages and B cells. There are two types of helper T cells: Th1 and Th2. Th1 stimulates cell-mediated immunity. When Th1 cells recognize a viral antigen, for example, they secrete cytokines (interleukin 2 IL-2, and interferon IFM) to signal killer T cells to lyse or penetrate and destroy infected cells.

Th2 stimulate humoral immunity. When they recognize antigens they produce cytokines (IL-4, 5 10) that stimulate B cells to produce antibodies including IgE. The antibodies then bind to specialised IgE receptors on the surfaces of mast cells, basophils and eosinophils in the bloodstream and connective tissue. These cells that contain allergy-inducing chemicals, such as histamine are present in the connective tissues, in the respiratory tract, gastrointestinal tract, urinary tract, nasal passages and skin. IgE antibodies can circulate in the bloodstream and become distributed on mast cells throughout the body. The allergic response begins when an allergen binds to IgE antibodies that are in turn bound to mast cells thereby activating the mast cells to degranulate and release their chemicals. Mast cell degranulation can result in vomiting, diarrhea, constriction of airways, coughing, sneezing, skin itch, a drop in blood pressure, and in severe cases, shock and death.[38]

In the Th1-Th2 paradigm, a balance of the two T cell functions was seen as crucial. Non-atopic people show mainly Th1 immunity characteristics. They produce interferon that inhibits the growth of the Th2 cells. Again, some doctors suggested that vaccination was upsetting this balance by stimulating the Th2 side to produce excessive numbers of antibodies and limiting the Th1 (which would result in symptoms of disease).[39]

There was evidence that childhood infections (with fever and malaise) were important in the development of a balanced immune system by 'teaching' the body how to handle other infections and that their vaccination-induced decline meant this developmental role was lacking.[40]

And yet too much vitamin D,[41] some suggested, or genetic predisposition, could just as easily cause the imbalance.

By 2003, the paradigm that compressed the immune processes into a tidy concept itself came under fire. The "dogma that Th1 and Th2 cells are associated with cell mediated and humoral immunity, respectively, has recently been reevaluated... It appears that the mechanism of protection involves a complex combination of antibody and T-cell responses..."[42] Such reevaluations suggested that antibody count – such as that of an IgE RAST test, as a measure of sensitivity to an allergen, or other antibodies, as a measure of vaccine efficacy – was just a small part of the total immune response.[43]

The rigid model could not accommodate new data.[44]

Age & year of birth

Age at which the allergy developed was identified as a significant risk factor. Toddlers, far more than adults developed the allergy. The year of birth, anyone born after about 1990 and depending on birth country, carried an increased risk.

The age of "onset" was the age at which the allergy was first discovered and not the moment of sensitization. Sensitization would have occurred before onset. According to the LEAP home page, the majority of allergic children had their first reaction to peanut between 14 and 24 months of age.

A review of pediatric peanut allergic patients at Johns Hopkins University indicated a median age of peanut exposure and reaction were 22 and 24 months respectively for children born between 1995 and 1997; for those born before 2000 the ages were 19 and 21 months; and for those born after 2000 their ages were 12 and 14 months.[45] The unusual ability to identify first exposure was anecdotal, using history and phone survey.

Year of birth was highly significant in the epidemic. ER records, cohort studies and eyewitness accounts as outlined in Chapter 1, showed that an acceleration of peanut allergy in children began around 1990. Children born in western countries had an increasing chance of developing the allergy. By 2009, children had an estimated 1 in 50 chance of developing the allergy.

Since adults rarely developed peanut allergy, the rising adult statistics for the allergy were misleading – as peanut allergic children aged their status was reflected in a new statistic. Children sensitized in 1990 were 19 in 2009.

Birth month

A correlation was discovered between the risk of developing severe allergy and the month of a child's birth. A study indicated that 55% of children born during Jan. through March had their first reactions to peanuts during those same months.[46] Similarly, 57% of children born in Oct. through Dec. experienced their first reactions during that three-month period. The same phenomenon was noted for those born between April and June.

The correlation prompted speculation that dietary changes on or near a child's first birthday could explain the trend.

A Netherlands study detected an increased risk of cow milk and egg allergies in patients born in Nov. through Jan. with a decrease in May. The same correlation was identified between period of birth and period of first peanut reaction.[47] In a study from Duke University, 31% of the peanut allergic patients were born in October through Dec., compared with 18% in April through June. This observation pointed to a possible relationship between environmental or seasonal factors but lack of data prevented further speculation.

Gender

The strong gender bias in the peanut allergy went unnoticed by researchers until the later 2000s. Its significance was little understood but echoed the same striking trend in autism. Prevalence of peanut allergy was higher in boys than girls – in a ratio greater than 2:1.

Of 140 patients at a Duke University pediatrics clinic (70 born between 1988 and 1999 and 70 born between 2000 and 2005) 66% of those that were allergic to peanuts were male.[48] In a FAAN on-line survey 67% of peanut allergic children respondents were male. Similarly, of a Johns Hopkins University group 63% were male. [49] Other studies supported this trend.[50] In an Australian 10 year survey of clinical consultation for food allergy in children under five, 60% were male.[51] A male predominance of peanut allergy was reported in children younger than 18 years – 1.7% vs. 0.7% between males and females.[52] Only one study, a US CDC report 2008, indicated that girls and boys were about even in prevalence of overall food allergy.

While there was no explanation for the disparity between peanut allergic boys and girls, a parallel phenomenon appeared in children with autism and Asperger's Syndrome.

Hans Asperger, who identified the Syndrome on the autism spectrum, originally believed that no girls were affected by the condition he described in 1944, although he later revised this conclusion. This gap was as high as 10:1 for Asperger's and 4:1 for autism. In 1964, Bernard Rimland observed that boys tended to be more vulnerable to "organic damage" than girls whether through hereditary disease, acquired infection or other conditions.

The rate of autism and peanut allergy in children increased within the same window of time starting around 1990 with a concomitant sex ratio difference. The rate of autism in the US was 1 in 1,000 after 1970. In 2009, it was believed to be about 1 in 100 children in the US.[53] Peanut allergy had no significant profile prior to 1990. By 2009, it appeared in about 1 in 50 children in the US and many other western countries.

Increasingly, the health of boys and the birth rate of boys has been impacted by environmental pollutants at a higher rate than girls. The global decline in male births was nowhere more evident than in the Aamjiwnaang First Nations community in Ontario, Canada. In this small population downriver of polluting petrochemical plants, female births outnumbered male births 2:1 in 2003.[54]

Race

Race was not seen to be a risk factor for developing peanut allergy.[55] However, geography, access to medical care, cultural norms, socio-economic and political factors can be associated with race. These factors may be reflected in the 2008 CDC National Health Interview Survey. In this survey, food allergy was reported in 3.1% of Hispanic children under 18 years of age. This is significantly different from non-Hispanic white and non-Hispanic black children of whom 4.1% and 4% respectively had food allergies.

One study asked whether minority children were being under-diagnosed or under-treated for allergic conditions or whether they truly had a lower incidence of such allergies.[56] This 2005 study found significant racial, ethnic, and socioeconomic differences in the prevalence of childhood allergic disorders, especially peanut or tree nut allergy, but only as it related to prescribed injectable epinephrine.

Food allergy reactions appeared to occur at a higher rate in Asian children living in westernized countries.[57] [58] One study found allergies in general to be higher in Asian than in European children in the UK.[59] In contrast, food allergy in Asian children living in China is traditionally low. Around 2005, however, this freedom from allergy changed when 1% of children living in Singapore and Hong Kong were found to be peanut allergic.

Mode of delivery and intestinal flora

Researchers suggested that a child born by cesarean section had an increased risk of developing allergies. They postulated that this mode of delivery used for one third of US children delayed the growth of important flora in newborn intestine thereby impacting the immune system. While they conceded that cesarean was not linked to any specific allergy, it appeared to intensify atopy.

A Norwegian study focused on birth by cesarean section, the use of antibiotics in creating dysbiosis (bacteria imbalance in the digestive system) and low levels of digestive flora as risk factors in reactions to egg, fish and nuts.

Among the 2,803 children whose mothers were atopic, birth through caesarean section was associated with a seven-fold increased risk of reactions to foods. The association between caesarean and food allergy was not significant in children of non-atopic mothers nor was maternal or infant use of antibiotics.[60] These conclusions were echoed by a German study.[61]

Cesarean delayed the colonization of flora in newborn intestine. Balanced intestinal bacteria were seen as important for digestive health and the integrity of the colon. If ill digested proteins managed to escape through those walls and enter the blood stream, allergies could result. A subsequent article offered, however, that rather than increasing the overall risk of food allergy cesarean simply made allergics worse.[62]

Yet another study from Finland found that allergic children had different fecal micro flora with less lactobacilli and bifidobacteria. Probiotic and prebiotic supplements were given to 1,223 children over five years. Less IgE associated atopy occurred in 24% of cesarean delivered children who took the supplements.[63]

Cesarean births in the US peaked at an average 24.7% of births in 1988 then steadily declined between 1989 and 1996 before increasing yet again.[64] While the WHO recommended a maximum of 15% of births by cesarean, the US rate in 2006 was 31.1%.[65] In the UK, the cesarean birth rate was 10% in 1980, 11% in 1990 and 22% in 2002. In Israel, the cesarean birth rate was 10.7% in the 1980s[66], 16% in 1999[67] and 17-18% in 2006.[68]

While UK and Israeli cesarean rates were roughly comparable, prevalence of peanut allergy was significantly higher in the UK than in Israel (2% vs. .17%). These figures were the inverse for sesame allergy in children. In Israel 1.2% children were allergic to cow's milk and sesame, followed by egg (2002, 2008).[69] [70] Sesame allergy in UK children in a 2005 study was low at .1%.[71] These differences could not be explained by mode of delivery.

Cesarean birth like so many other factors appeared in general to exacerbate a tendency to allergy. But there was no specific link to the peanut allergy.

Maternal age at delivery

Since the average age of first time mothers had gradually increased doctors wondered whether if it was a risk factor for allergy in children. As with many of the proffered general risk factors, it failed to shed light on the peanut allergy.

An American study of 55 severely food allergic children sought to evaluate whether maternal age at birth was higher for children with IgE-mediated food allergy than for those without.[72] The mean maternal age at birth of children with food allergies was 31.2 years compared to the mean maternal age at birth of children without food allergies, 29.2 years. Mothers of children with a food allergy had 2.88 times greater odds of being aged <30 years at the time of delivery compared to control patients; 78% compared to 55%.

While an explanation for this disparity was not ventured in the study, environmental factors may have contributed. According to the CDC statistics, there was a greater tendency for older mothers 30+ to have cesarean.[73] This mode of delivery was shown to exacerbate atopy in children born to atopic mothers. Again, though, there was no connection between maternal age and the puzzling features of the peanut allergy – including its epidemic acceleration after 1990.

Socio-economic status

The destruction of the Berlin wall in 1989 and the fall of communism offered an opportunity for allergy researchers to better understand the divergent allergy trends in the two halves of the city.

People in the less affluent East Berlin had a significantly lower prevalence of atopic conditions than people living in the wealthier West. Within 10 years of reunification, however, a study of children indicated that the two halves had become the same in this regard. With reunification, researchers concluded, there came greater access to westernized health care and lifestyle. Cleaning products, antibiotics and other amenities had generally altered conditions for children born in the East and contributed to the increase in allergy.

Between 2003 and 2006, the German Health Interview and Examination Survey for Children and Adolescents collected information on asthma, atopic dermatitis, hay fever, and eczema for 17,641 children aged 1 to 17. The survey revealed that there was increased sensitization to 20 common allergens.[74]

A loss of disease burden with improved socio-economic conditions was presumed to have caused a dysregulation in the immune systems of children.[75] However, it seemed unlikely that in just 10 years, East Berlin would have become sufficiently germ reduced and affluent to have prompted such a significant increase in atopy. This abrupt development suggested a more immediate and invasive cause.

Nevertheless, the westernization of East Berlin did not explain the specificity of the peanut. In fact, peanut allergy appeared to be low for children in Berlin, East and West.[76] In a randomly selected population based survey of children in Berlin, the food allergens most commonly identified by oral challenge were apple, hazelnuts, soy, kiwi, carrot and wheat. 4.2% of children showed food allergy symptoms although no anaphylaxis. All reactions were mild and mainly due to pollen cross-associated food allergy. In this study, peanut was not an issue. However, in a 2005 analysis of physician reported cases of 103 anaphylactic children in Germany, foods were the most frequent cause of the reaction (57%, and 20% to peanut of this number) followed by insect stings (13%) and immunotherapy injections (12%). Peanuts and tree nuts were the foods most frequently causing the reactions.[77]

The description of this risk factor, however, stopped short of delineating the specific features of socio-economic status that were altered in East Berlin starting in 1989. The specific conditions that gave rise to peanut allergy elsewhere were presumably largely absent from East Berlin at this time. Given that prevalence of the peanut allergy was still low ten years after reunification, those conditions may have continued to exist to some degree.

Other research noted a connection between socio-economic status and prevalence of anaphylaxis in the UK.[78] Researchers used a map to highlight the more affluent areas of the country in which there was a slightly higher prevalence of anaphylaxis by virtue of ER admissions. Of these, reactions to drugs constituted over 50% of recorded triggers and food made up almost 20%; children under five made up the majority of these patients.

And yet, another UK study published in 2003 based on a longitudinal study in Avon, saw no statistically significant associations between peanut allergy and any socioeconomic factor.[79]

Large head circumference

Researchers seemed to reach the bottom of the barrel in 1999 when they correlated rise in allergy in children with the size of their heads.

A study of newborn cord blood samples and measurements revealed an increase in IgE related to large head circumference.[80] IgE does not cross the placenta and so was associated with the mother. However, it was used as an indication of future allergic tendency in the child.

The explanation for the relationship between a large head at birth and future allergy was curious. In affluent societies where nutrition is generally good, researchers explained, the fetus will grow rapidly during the early stages of pregnancy and will remain programmed to grow at this rate.[81] As the pregnancy progresses, the child will have a high nutrient demand which is difficult to meet. In a poor community with poor nutrition, the fetus is programmed to grow slowly and have lower nutrient demand. The high demand fetus is suddenly in a position where nutrient delivery is constant and therefore does not sustain growth. The brain and head continue to grow at the expense of the body that results in a big head and normal birth weight but poor nutrient delivery to other parts of the body. This in turn modifies the immune system. Apparently, the Th1 side is more susceptible to being switched off in adverse circumstances than Th2. Thus, it was suggested, the relationship of large head and suppressed Th1 side explained the increase in allergy in affluent societies.

While having a large head at birth may point to future allergies, according to limited studies, it did not point specifically at peanut.

Heredity

A broadly accepted risk factor in the development of allergy in children is heredity. While statistics revealed common allergy threads between siblings and mothers, again, this risk did not fit with the simple facts of the peanut allergy – its abrupt emergence around 1990 and its rapid spread. Genes do not change that quickly.

In 1996, it was observed that peanut allergy was more common in siblings of people with peanut allergy than in the parents or the general population.[82]

The higher rate of peanut allergy in the siblings of people with peanut allergy compared with the general population was about 7% vs. 1.3% in one study.[83] Peanut allergy was reported by 0.1% (3/2409) of grandparents, 0.6% (7/1213) of aunts and uncles, 1.6% (19/1218) of parents,[84] and 6.9% (42/610) of siblings according to a 1996 study.[85] In 2000, one researcher performed a study of monozygotic and dizygotic twins aged one to 58 in which one of the pair had the peanut allergy. Skin tests performed suggested that because more non-reactive monozygotic pairs had a positive test, than dizygotic pairs that there was a genetic influence on peanut allergy.[86]

This study defaulted to the idea that there may be an "allergy gene" that condemned some families to allergy.[87] It avoided discussion of differences between the twins as individuals with different medical experiences, gender, history, digestive health, kidney function and abilities to detoxify waste.

The same differences may have been at play in a provocative study using different strains of genetically engineered mice. The study showed that injections of peanut induced anaphylaxis in some but not all strains.[88] After vaccination with peanut, the mice were injected again three or five weeks later. Researchers were unable to induce anaphylaxis in two strains of albino mice AKR/J and BALB/c – neither IgE or IgG1 were found in these two strains although IgG2a was increased. Anaphylaxis was easily induced in the grey-brown C3H/HeSn strain.

A general genetic explanation was offered for these differences that, researchers proposed, might also exist in humans.

This vision of DNA was formulated by Francis Crick, who together with James Watson deciphered the structure of the DNA molecule in 1953. Crick came to believe that DNA controls life, an ubiquitous concept that is usually accepted as incontrovertible fact.

While moderate doctors such as Kenneth Bock suggested, "genetics may load the gun but environment pulls the trigger,"[89] a new generation of scientists have rejected the Crick DNA dogma outright. Genetics did not load the gun, environment did through the new concept of "epigenetics".

Cell biologist Dr. Bruce Lipton in his research at Stanford University School of Medicine in the early 1990s suggested that the environment, operating energetically through the membrane of the cells, actually controls the behavior and physiology of cells. In other words, the human body is not a biochemical machine at the mercy of self-actualizing genes (turn themselves on and off) but rather environment and the individual's perception of it control gene activity. Cells possess the ability to reprogram their own DNA as they are affected by diet, chronic thoughts and even vaccination. Such rewriting accounts for up to 98% of evolutionary transformation. In short, epigenetics suggested that people are masters of their own biology.

If this were true, there would be implications for a broader understanding of peanut allergy and perhaps also how to recover from it.

The traditional understanding of genetics, however, cannot explain the peanut allergy epidemic. Hundreds of thousands of children would have had to experience a simultaneous change in their genetic profile starting around 1990 and occurring regularly since then to account for the current peanut allergy phenomenon. This would have been highly unlikely.

Immune system overload

The 4 A's — allergy, autism, ADHD and asthma — have emerged from fundamental dysfunctions in nutritional, immune and inflammatory factors, suggested Ken Bock in *Healing the New Childhood Epidemics* (2007).[90] Contributing to these unhealthy conditions in many children were: fungal overgrowth especially Candida that has spread from the gut; poor diet and eating habits; and deficiencies in probiotics (beneficial digestive flora), essential fatty acids, stomach acid and digestive enzymes. Further crippling a child's immune system were antibiotic overuse and childhood vaccinations.

If a robust Th1 side immune response is not established, Bock offered, a child can develop a chronic low-grade infection from an injected vaccine antigen, such as measles. Such an infection can linger in the gut resulting in inflammation, which in turn sends out immune cell messengers, cytokines, that trigger even more inflammation in distant parts of the body. This can lead to inflammation in joints, the lining of the gastrointestinal tract and even the brain. All inflammation contributes to allergies, stated Bock. And allergies cause even more inflammation.

While these overlapping factors contributed to the prevalence of the 4-As, the "smoking gun" that explained the specificity and sudden prevalence of peanut allergy had yet to be unearthed.

Vaccination

Bock (2007) pointed to the mercury preservative Thimerosal in vaccines as a significant factor in the epidemics of autism, ADHD, asthma and allergies in children. He also expressed concern over the increase in number of vaccines, the multi-dose single shots, undetected health conditions of the child at the time of vaccination, and more.[91]

For scientists, it was difficult to confirm the role of vaccination because there were no studies of non-vaccinated populations in the US – there were so few children who have not been vaccinated. According to the CDC, US vaccination rates have been at record highs. While 77% of US kids met all vaccination goals in 2007 at least 90% met the goal for each vaccine except for DTaP but even those kids received three out of the four recommended doses.[92]

Recognizing that there was a significant gap in medicine's understanding of vaccination outcomes, two Members of US Congress introduced the "Comprehensive Comparative Study of Vaccinated and Unvaccinated Populations Act" in 2007. This Bill was slow to achieve support but was to be reintroduced to the 111th Congress in 2009.[93]

It was left to a Grade 9 Connecticut student Devi Lockwood[94] to conduct an ad hoc study of the few non-vaccinated populations in the US in 2007. Devi looked at the Old Order Amish who discouraged vaccination. In these communities, peanut allergy was virtually non-existent. But because the Amish communities were genetically connected, their example in understanding the role of vaccination in allergy was rejected by the CDC.[95]

And so, Devi turned to Vashon Island, WA, a haven for alternative medicine where 1,600 school-aged children were unvaccinated. Devi looked at two schools, elementary and middle, with high exemption rates on Vashon Island and two similar schools in his hometown of Ridgefield that had a low exemption rates. Where the vaccination rate was high the prevalence of peanut allergy increased significantly. Where vaccination rate was low, so too was the prevalence of the allergy. At the two Vashon schools there were three peanut allergic children. In Ridgefield, there were 22 at the two schools. All peanut allergic children had been vaccinated.

Significantly, there were no un-vaccinated children with peanut allergy in this small study.

Risks associated with vaccination were infrequently ventured in medical literature through the 1990s although increasing in the later 2000s. Vaccination, an event shared by the vast majority of western children, carried clear political, social and economic implications. Doctors would not want to dissuade the public from getting their shots. The connection between allergy and vaccination was not new. And yet, vaccination did not appear to be a primary concern within the plethora of research. As already noted, as a potential means of causing atopy vaccination was lumped together with every other risk factor within the broad shouldered Th1-Th2 paradigm.

"Outgrowing" peanut allergy

No one knew how or why a child "outgrew" a peanut allergy. And even when a child did, this resolution of the allergy was not always permanent.

Statistics reported in 2001 indicated that as many as 22% of peanut allergic children developed tolerance to the food later in life.[96] Chances of outgrowing the allergy were improved if the child had low levels of peanut-specific serum IgE antibodies in infancy (less than 5kU per liter).[97]

A 1998 study of 15 children compared those who had outgrown their clinical reactivity to peanut and those who had not. All children "resolvers" and "persisters" had reacted to peanut first at the age of about 11 months and they were re-tested at about age five.

Although in skin prick tests, resolvers had much smaller wheals, blood tests showed that the IgE total and peanut specific levels between the two groups did not differ.[98] Allergy to other foods was less common in resolvers (2/15) than persisters (9/15).

In a phone follow up two years later with the resolvers in this study, only one had reacted by vomiting after eating peanut. A note of caution no doubt accompanied the news of this apparent resolution, however, since some children previously thought to have outgrown the allergy have reverted.[99] [100]

An unusual case was reported in 2005 of a child whose peanut allergy resolved following a bone marrow transplant.[101] In this instance, not only was a food challenge negative but also specific IgE to peanut was found to be undetectable (<0.35 KU A).

Summary of Risk Factors

The frantic attempts to find common ground between the hundreds of thousands of peanut allergic children as the 1990s unfolded revealed a profound level of confusion. Intense study had been made into peanut consumption, the role of atopy and socio-economic status leaving researchers with more questions than answers. And despite the preponderance of research, significant risk factors such as gender and vaccination were given little or no attention.

Deepening the concern of perplexed doctors was the unanticipated spread of the allergy into China and Africa through the 2000s. Many had bet their reputations on the idea that just eating peanuts was a primary risk for developing the allergy and that boiling peanuts had protected the Chinese from it.

What emerged from the tangle of research ultimately was a partial profile of the person most at risk for developing the allergy: a toddler (male 2:1) born after 1990 in a western country and whose ability to detoxify had been impaired by environmental factors. These factors appeared to include vaccination but such a proposal amounted to a hypothesis very much at odds with official medical explanations for the phenomenal rise in allergy in the 20th century.

Chapter 3

Theories

By 2000, doctors had matched general risk factors with clinical observations to produce several explanations for the general rise in allergy. Each disparate theory, however, was a bad fit for the peanut allergy. None could adequately explain its sudden and simultaneous emergence in western countries and its almost exclusive rise in children.

Theories applied to the peanut allergy included the Broken Skin Hypothesis, the Ingestion Hypothesis, the Helminth Hypothesis and the Hygiene Hypothesis. Fundamental to each of these was a definition of allergy as a "genetically determined disorder".[1] Each assumed that allergy is an inherited dysregulation of the immune system that leads to an elevated production of IgE antibodies in response to protein allergens.[2][3] And as such, if the environment contributes to a child's allergy it merely unmasks an extant predisposition to reactivity. Genetics loads the gun and the environment fires it. Humans are fated to allergy.

The Toxin Hypothesis, developed before the peanut allergy epidemic emerged, provided a lone counter point to the official hypotheses. This hypothesis was alone in its proposal that allergy is not a dysfunction at all. Within this new concept, allergy serves a purpose as an evolved immune defense against acute toxicity. Whether sensitized to toxic proteins by inhalation, broken skin, injection or consumption, the purpose of the allergic response is to eject the toxic threat from the body as fast as possible. The idea that this dangerous reaction may have a designed purpose was an important clue that doctors had either missed or dismissed.

Indeed, at the end of the day a kind of medical myopia appeared to constrain the perspective of many researchers. Few were motivated to look for clues outside of the immediate specimens of child or peanut. American microbiologist René Dubos had observed that it is seldom recognized that each society and every civilization creates its own diseases.[4] If this was true, then a broad framework of investigation that embraced other areas of thought including history could be required to drag the solution into public consciousness.

Broken Skin Hypothesis

It was proposed in a 2003 study that exposure to low doses of peanut proteins through broken and inflamed skin had caused mass allergic sensitization.[5] Researchers were surprised to find that many eczema ointments commonly used on children contained refined peanut oil. An analysis of the oil revealed that there were enough intact proteins to sensitize atopic children to peanuts. This, they suggested, was the source of the epidemic.

Data was used from the Avon Longitudinal Study of Parents and Children, a geographically defined cohort study in southwest England of 13,971 preschool children. In this group, there were 49 children confirmed to have an allergy to peanut. Questionnaires, medical records, biologic samples including cord blood provided information on children born in 1991 and 1992 up to the age of about three years. Of significance was their belief that sensitization to peanut occurred after birth.

To explain the allergy to peanut, researchers developed a somewhat convoluted theory based on two risk factors. The first was that there was a strong association between eczema caused by an intolerance to cow's milk and peanut allergy. Although none asked what had caused the milk allergy, it was a problem because mothers then switched their children from milk to a soya beverage. This decision became the real risk factor, they argued, because it would have sensitized the children to soya proteins that are similar to those of peanut. Curiously, none of the peanut allergic children appeared to be reactive to soya – they could consume it without apparent concern.

Nevertheless, once sensitized ostensibly to soya, peanut entered the scenario via a second risk factor – refined peanut oil in skin ointments[6] that was applied to the oozing, inflamed eczema (dairy must then not have been the only cause of eczema because it had been removed from the diet).

The oil in the skin ointments was alleged to be free of sensitizing peanut protein. However, researchers analyzed the oil and found that it contained enough protein to produce "positive responses in leukocyte histamine-release assays in such patients."[7] Additional studies in 2005 supported this idea concluding that epicutaneous exposure to peanut protein could cause oral intolerance in experiments with mice.[8]

And yet, an equal number of atopic children with eczema did not develop peanut allergy. This gave rise to doubts that therapeutic pharmaceutical products containing refined peanut oil played a role in sensitization.[9]

Scanning back in time, crude peanut oil loaded with the dangerous proteins had been used on skin with cuts and abrasions for decades without incident. The health benefits of rubbing peanut oil on skin was recommended by agricultural chemist George Washington Carver (1864-1943) to help heal polio. Carver was certain that peanut oil applied during a massage not only saturated the skin and flesh but also actually entered the blood stream and helped restore life to limbs withered by polio. In 1933 the Associated Press carried a story about Carver's alleged successes with polio peanut oil massages and, for a time, his Alabama school resembled a pilgrimage site.

Thousands of Americans including President Roosevelt (elected in 1932) who visited Carver in 1938 enjoyed a peanut oil rub down. Doctors recommended and developed their own brand such as the "Vitalized Peanut Oil" in the fall of 1934. Not to be outdone, another skin oil entrepreneur, the Rose Miller Company sought approval from the FDA for its peanut oil "bust developer".[10]

Casting more doubt on the Broken Skin Hypothesis was the fact that the use of peanut oil in ointments for eczema and other skin conditions had been constant for decades. There was no sudden acceleration of use that would have coincided with the abrupt surge of peanut allergic children around 1990. As well, the eczema ointments used on atopic children would certainly have contained other oils and ingredients to which the children did not appear to be sensitized. Why the peanut epidemic as opposed to other potentially cross reactive food ingredients such as corn, safflower or indeed cottonseed?

The use of peanut oil, refined or not, in skin creams does not explain the epidemic proportions of this allergy. It does, however, open questions on the use of refined peanut oil in other potential methods of sensitization such as in medicines consumed orally or through injection.

The relative allergenicity of this peanut oil did not worry the US Food and Drug Administration, however. The FDA had given refined peanut oil GRAS status (generally recognized as safe). GRAS indicates that its use in food is presumed safe based either on a history of use before 1958 or on published scientific evidence. A manufacturer does not need approval by the FDA to use the oil in foods.[11] And yet, in 1998, researchers confirmed that refined peanut oil did contain trace proteins that were the same as those in crude peanut oil.[12] [13] The FDA at their web site acknowledged the studies and observed that the levels of peanut protein varied due to differences in refining processes and the detection method used. According to this agency "most highly refined oils contained 0.2-2.2 µg/ml of protein".[14] But, again, it was not a concern.

Nut and seed oil refiners Welch, Holme & Clark Co. published a web page on "Refined Peanut Oil N.F."[15] N.F. stands for National Formulary from the U.S. Pharmacopeia (USP). The N.F. is a book of public pharmacopeial standards for medicines, excipients and other mixtures. In it is a procedure for refining peanut oil.[16] According to the Welch, Holme & Clark site, "high quality" peanut oil is extremely difficult to obtain because almost all refined peanut oil contains traces of cottonseed oil – even in small quantities the presence of cottonseed oil violates the specifications of the USP.

There being a "high quality" refined peanut oil implied that there were those of low quality. To that end, the WHO Codex Alimentarius Committee on Food Labeling resisted giving its full endorsement to the oil in 2000.[17] While DBPC tests in which peanut allergic volunteers consumed refined peanut oil without reaction, the WHO questioned the refining processes and lack of thorough data and even the quality and validity of the analytical procedures used to determine the concentration of residual protein in the oils.

Ultimately, instead of investigating the allergenicity of the oil further, the WHO committee relied on the oil's history of previous use and concluded that the inclusion of refined peanut oil in foods did not have to be revealed to consumers.[18] There were two allergenic foods that did not need to be labeled: refined peanut oil and refined soya bean oil. In US made foods the oil was still not labeled in 2009.

And yet, children have been sensitized to refined peanut oil contained in oral vitamin D supplements.[19] And the peanut oil used in baby formula had caused anaphylaxis in infants sensitized to peanut.[20] Some doctors argued that peanut oil should be excluded from medications altogether or at least listed as an ingredient.[21] [22]

While doctors remained divided on the allergenicity of refined peanut oil in foods, skin creams and oral medications, it seemed beyond the bounds of discussion to review its use in injected medicines. There appeared to be not one published investigation into this route of sensitization. And yet, the refined peanut oil described for use in foods that had sensitized some children was the same oil used in medical injections. At the Welch, Holme & Clark web site was a declaration that their refined peanut oil "fully meets U.S.P. specifications in every respect and is suitable for injectable use."[23]

Ingestion Hypothesis

Researchers seemed to think that by pin pointing how and when children first ate peanut they could stop the epidemic. It was presumed that just eating peanut could result in sensitization if a child had a compromised digestive system. Alternatively, genetics contributed to sensitization if the child had an inherent dysregulation of the Th1-Th2 paradigm. In this hypothesis, there was no specific mechanism of sensitization to peanut. The allergic individual was assumed to have a tendency to capricious sensitization. And the fact that peanut was so allergenic only increased the chances of becoming sensitized to it.

While the theory of ingestion was obvious and easy to comprehend, as an explanation for an epidemic of food allergy it did not fit. Although allergists have stated, "ostensibly, ingestion of peanut is the sensitizing route,"[24] ingestion was not found to be a risk factor for the allergy in its epidemic proportions. As reviewed in Chapter 2, many studies indicated that ingestion of peanut – early or later in life, boiled, roasted or refined, in breast milk or nipple creams, in small or large quantities – had no apparent relevance in the epidemic.

In addition, it was implausible that hundreds of thousands of children had become allergic to this one food in the space of just 20 years by ingestion alone. The hypothesis proposed that all peanut allergic children (an average of 90,960 US children a year between 1997 and 2002 reaching 871,200 peanut allergic children under 18 in 2002[25]) had weakened digestive abilities or a Th2 skewed system, or both. The large numbers alone were just too great to sustain this explanation.

And so, puzzled doctors moved their attention away from the allergic child to examine the peanut itself. One mystified doctor opined that there "appears to be something unique about the peanut that is not shared by other members of the legume family or most other food proteins."[26]

In analyzing what appeared to make some foods more allergenic than others researchers focused on three aspects of their proteins: size; abundance; and stability.[27]

Proteins are made of strings of amino acids called epitopes. A minimum size epitope of about 30 amino acids with a molecular weight of 3 kD is required for a protein to cross-link IgE antibodies on the surface of mast cells. If a protein is less than that, it is unable to cross-link IgE and an allergic response will not result. Peanut proteins (Ara h 1 and Ara h 2) and the soya bean proteins (Gly m 1) have many allergenic epitopes and many IgE binding sites that allow them to cross-link IgE on the surface of mast cells very efficiently. The molecular weight of peanut varies but Ara h 1 was noted to have a molecular weight of between 20 and 63.5 kDa and Ara h 2 to have a weight of 17kDa.[28] [29]

Peanut proteins are also resistant to degradation by stomach acid and enzymes in the gastrointestinal tract. The "hydrophobic" residues of the amino acids in Ara h

1 peanut epitope, for example, are protected from digestion within the structure of the epitope.[30] Nuts and seeds are difficult to digest.

Another "allergenic" feature of proteins is their stability when heated or processed (grinding and cooking). One study claimed that the reason peanut allergy was not seen in China was that people there boil or fry peanuts which lowers the quantity of Ara h 1 in the peanut (although not its ability to bind to IgE). And compared to dry roasting that was used extensively in the US, these methods of preparation resulted in a lower level of IgE binding to Ara h 2 and 3. In addition, the high temperature of dry roasting appears to increase the allergenicity of the proteins.[31] [32] According to one researcher, the peanut has adjuvant properties that make it "a perfect allergen".[33]

And consuming a certain protein in a concentrated form may enhance the risk of developing an allergy to it. For example, ovalbumin and ovomucoid that are the two major allergens in chicken egg represent 54% and 11% of the total protein, respectively. Ara h 1 makes up about 16% of the total 24-29% protein of a peanut.[34]

Despite the widely acknowledged allergenicity of peanuts, Americans had been consuming this dietary staple for decades without apparent concern. And given that the allergenicity of peanuts is the same the world over, it could not be used to explain epidemiological features of the allergy – why some countries but not others. Researchers concluded, for example, that the divergent prevalence of the allergy in the UK compared to Israel "is not accounted for by differences in atopy, social class, genetic background, or peanut allergenicity."[35] Allergenicity, high or low consumption, age of first introduction, all appeared to have little or no bearing on the absence of peanut allergy in Russia and India and recent emergence in Hong Kong and Singapore in 2007.

A valuable clue existed in the fact of the allergy's sudden emergence around 1990. Something in the lives of children changed at that time that persisted and even worsened through the 2000s – whatever it was, though, it seemed to have little to do with eating peanuts.

Toxin Hypothesis

First proposed in 1991 by biologist Margie Profet (b. 1958) the Toxin Hypothesis provided an alternative framework for understanding allergy. It provided for the first time, a purpose for this disturbing immune response.

IgE is a universal antibody that was programmed millions of years ago. It appears in mammals, marsupials, and non-mammals including fish and frogs.[36] The evolutionary age of IgE mediated allergy may be more than 60 million years. Its persistence in spite of or because of its damaging effects on the body must have an evolved purpose, argued Profet.

Profet suggested that allergy evolved in mammals as a "last line of defense against toxic substances in the environment in the form of secondary plant compounds and venoms."[37]

Because toxins are ubiquitous, humans have developed a variety of tactics to defend against them whether they are inhaled, consumed, rubbed on the skin or injected (ie. bee venom). These include the senses of smell and sight, remembering and avoiding, eating a diversity of foods, peeling fruits and vegetables, cooking foods, enzymatic destruction and shedding epithelial surfaces of organs regularly exposed to toxins, such as in the gut, lungs and skin.

However, when these primary defenses have previously been unable to stop a specific toxin from entering the blood stream, allergy is created. The defense tactics of allergy are designed to expel this toxin as quickly as possible from the body.

The chemicals released during an IgE mediated allergic response can result in vomiting, diarrhea, itching, sneezing, tearing, bronchial constriction and coughing. These are all ways in which the body is able to expel toxins from the body. The decrease in blood pressure that slows blood flow is an attempt to protect internal organs from potentially circulating toxins.

Profet suggested that nontoxic proteins that become allergens such as peanut are either "reliable correlates" of toxins or carriers of toxins. For example, aflatoxin from mold spores often contaminates peanuts. Allergy to peanuts may actually represent an IgE response to the aflatoxin and, secondarily, to the peanut proteins associated with it.[38] In several allergy studies, mice were made allergic by inhaling or eating peanut mixed with a bacterium – cholera.[39]

To create allergy, the body must covalently bind substances (toxin or carrier or both) to serum proteins.

Valency is characterized by the sharing of electrons in a chemical compound; the number of pairs of electrons an atom can share. A valence is an electron ring that encircles the atom. The first ring or valence of any atom can only hold two electrons. The second valence only holds eight. For example, Hydrogen has just one valence with one electron and is always looking for a second. Because it is looking to complete its valence it is reactive and unstable, liable to bind to other elements that are also looking to complete their valence. Oxygen with six electrons in its second valence will bind well to two hydrogen molecules. Together they complete the valence of the other by sharing electrons. Oxygen shares two electrons from the two hydrogen molecules and each of these shares one from the oxygen molecule. These two elements are co-valently bound in a very stable molecule known as water.

Molecules liable to bind more readily with blood serum are those with low molecular weight. Researchers have pointed to the low weight of drugs that must bind to carrier proteins in the body to elicit sensitization (less than 1,000 Da) whereas high molecular weight molecules (larger than 5,000 Da) can act as complete antigens or bind covalently.[40]

The weight of a molecule, measured in Daltons (Da), is the sum of the weights of the atoms (including electrons and protons) of which it is made. For example, the molecular weight of water is 18 Daltons. The molecular weight of the peanut Ara h 1 protein is between 69,000 and 63,500 Daltons or 63.5 kDa. Human IgE antibodies have reacted to three epitopes or strings of amino acids in this protein.[41] Ara h 2 has a molecular weight of 17 kDa. Human IgE identified two binding epitopes in this protein. The approximate molecular weights of peanut have been identified: Ara h 3 is about 60 kDa; Ara h 4, 37 kDa; Ara h 5, 15 kDa; Ara h 6, 15 kDa; Ara h 7, 15 kDa; and Ara h 8, 15 kDa.[42]

If the bond between blood serum protein and hapten (a small molecule that can elicit an immune response only when bound to the carrier like a toxin) or carrier is covalent, it is strong and the kidneys cannot filter the hapten. It will continue to circulate in the blood allowing the immune system to form antibodies to it. A covalent bond between hapten and carrier protein is usually a requirement for the creation of IgE to the hapten.

Proteins that are especially efficient carriers of a wide spectrum of toxic haptens – for example, proteins with hydrophobic pockets that readily bind lipophilic substances, as is the case with the peanut protein – may be the most common targets of IgE antibodies.

But food allergy is not always so linear, Profet reminded readers. It is a complex process by which even two foods consumed together can become linked in the digestive tract if one binds to the toxic hapten of another.[43]

> If allergy is designed to defend against toxins that
> evade enzymatic detoxification, allergic susceptibility
> to drugs and ability to detoxify drugs are expected to
> be inversely related.[44]

In explaining why allergies are more prevalent in industrial societies compared to foraging societies, Profet pointed to exposure over sustained periods to a range of hidden toxins such as food additives or chemicals in soaps and skin creams. These toxins are hard to avoid using general immune defenses. Making matters worse in industrialized society, crowded conditions result in a greater number of respiratory infections that in turn are known to increase IgE levels, suggested Profet. This increases allergic sensitivity to the environment.[45]

In contrast, the Hygiene Hypothesis (below) proposed that the tendency to develop allergies is due to insufficient natural exposure to pathogens rather than an excess exposure. Industrialized societies are protected unnaturally by anti-bacterial products and drugs and vaccines. In these societies, people are unable to mount a proper immune defense to viral or bacterial pathogen thereby disrupting the Th1-Th2 paradigm. The body favors Th2 that stimulates the production of antibodies including IgE.

At the time of Profet's writing in 1991 the peanut allergy appeared to be just one of a widening range of allergies in western societies. Since then, no one has picked up the Toxin Hypothesis and applied it more specifically to the peanut allergy epidemic in children. Fine tuning Profet's generalized thesis, perhaps the answer to the specific features of the peanut allergy could have been better understood by unearthing: which toxins other than aflatoxin were associated with peanut; whether there were any proteins correlated to or homologous with peanut to which children were being exposed; and which defense systems were failing first or worst when it came to peanut. How were these associated toxins or correlates with peanut accessing the body?

Helminths Hypothesis

Helminths are parasitic worms that live in the human body. It surprised researchers in the 1980s to discover that people heavily infected with certain worms had few allergies. Neil Lynch at the University of Venezuela showed that 90% of Venezuelan Indians living in the rainforest had worms but no allergies. 10% of rich Venezuelans living in the cities had only light worm infections and 43% had allergies. Similar studies confirmed this feature of certain helminths. An Ethiopian study showed that people infected with hookworm, have a low frequency of asthma.[46] A study of helminth-infected Gabonese children showed that a parasite-specific IL10 response in the host suppressed atopy.[47]

From this general "worms vs. wealth" concept researchers developed an explanation for all allergies: because parasites and humans have co-evolved, they have a symbiotic relationship in which helminths "protect" humans from developing immune-mediated diseases (colitis, diabetes, etc.) and allergy.[48] According to the theory, while allergy evolved in humans in order to expel helminths, the worms had their own defenses in turn that suppressed the human response. However, in the west, hygienic conditions using pesticides and sanitation protocols had largely eliminated helminths from the human population. And without the historic presence of worms, humans were left open to random allergic symptoms.

There are two general categories of helminths: round worms (ascaris, hookworms, trichinella, filarial and eye worms); and flat worms (tape worm, fluke). These worms bury into or latch onto the intestinal wall of their hosts where they feed on blood, cells and tissue fluids. They lay eggs and reproduce easily. A heavy infection of helminths will lead to their spread from the digestive system into other areas of the body.

But the lack of helminths in the west, again, had left the immune systems of hundreds of thousands of people unbalanced and predictably dysfunctional. Without the suppressing effects of helminths, suggested some researchers, the drive towards the Th2-allergy inducing side of the immune system is so strong that "bystander proteins" become easy targets for IgE antibodies.[49] The Helminth Hypothesis explained that without enough parasitic worms in their intestinal tracts, humans are doomed to acquire bowel disease, autoimmune conditions and allergies.

Identifying this doctor-approved concept as a market opportunity, pharmaceutical companies moved quickly to develop the first worm-based "vaccine" for food allergy.[50] Western doctors also began to offer, "worm therapy" to modulate the immune systems of desperate allergy sufferers. The treatment consisted of a deliberate dose of eggs from the pig whipworm, Trichuris suis Ova (TSO).[51]

But while certain helminth infections can reduce severity of allergic response, additional research indicates that they do not appear to prevent the production of IgE antibodies to any number of allergens. The apparent value of a heavy helminth infection is in making the infected person hypo-reactive.[52] For example, where low concentrates of dust mites produced reactions in Dutch subjects, Gabonese children (infected with schistosome) with high IgE to mites needed extremely high concentrations of the allergen before mast cell degranulation was seen.[53]

In fact, extremely high levels of IgE accompany helminth infections. However, much of the IgE was rarely linked to the helminths themselves because, it was suggested, they were efficient at cloaking themselves.[54] Therefore, this mass of IgE was generally believed to be "non specific". This mysterious flood of non-specific antibodies, some researchers offered, prevented mast cell or basophil degranulation by filling up their binding sites. This left little room for additional specific antibodies.[55]

And yet, "if allergy had evolved primarily to protect against helminths, it would represent astonishingly poor design by natural selection."[56] Margie Profet suggested in her research that many of the allegedly "non-specific" IgE antibodies were actually specific to the excretions and secretions of the helminths that contained toxins absorbed from the host's diet. Helminths produce toxins from which African children with heavy infections have suddenly died.[57] [58]

The Helminth Hypothesis had other flaws. It could not account for the many phenomena of allergy including why blood pressure drops during a strong allergic response nor why these responses are potentially lethal. Anticoagulants released during allergic reactions appear to have no purpose in defense against helminths. Heparin, however, inhibits the procoagulants of certain snake and insect venoms that fit with the Toxin Hypothesis. If allergy had evolved to protect against helminths, it made no adaptive sense to Profet.

It seemed unlikely that without worms humans would malfunction – there were millions of people without worms who were equally without Crohn's or ulcerative colitis or allergies. In addition, studies indicated that worms were not the only presence that could suppress allergic reactivity. An infection of Helicobacter pylori bacteria was known to dampen allergies. Doctors also suggested that a decreasing prevalence of H. pylori in children of industrialized countries might be associated with the epidemics of asthma and allergy.[59]

In the end, it seemed more likely that the complete suppression of the immune system by helminths was not symbiotic but rather a straightforward manipulation of the host whose defenses had been neutralized to the advantage of the parasites.

Unchecked, a helminth infection will destroy health and shorten life. The body can produce hydatid cysts containing other cysts and tapeworm heads known as hydatid sand. If a human ingests a hydatid egg, a cyst will develop somewhere in the body. These cysts must be very carefully removed by surgery. If the cyst is punctured and the contents spill into the body, anaphylaxis can occur[60] and each daughter cyst will then mature into additional cysts.

Heavy helminth infections will cause nutritional deficiency, bowel obstruction, appendicitis and peritonitis, anemia, vomiting, internal bleeding, abdominal pain, diarrhea, anorexia, eosinophilia. The pork tapeworm taenia solium can enter the brain leading to seizures and cysticercosis, parasitic infestation of the central nervous system. For health reasons, some religions have historically forbidden pork consumption.

The host's lymphatic system is also heavily taxed the longer helminths propagate. Their toxic secretions are released into the intestines to be absorbed by the host's bloodstream. This phenomenon makes the host susceptible to viral and bacterial infections.

Ill effects slowly overwhelm a human with a heavy helminth infection. In the meantime, the successful parasite through the fecal matter of the infected person spreads its eggs to other hosts through contaminated water, soil, contact and food. The spread of worms is enhanced in a society that is poverty stricken, badly nourished, stationary (the people are not foragers) and has lost the knowledge of how to manage parasitic infections through natural means. The inflammation that the helminths suppress is caused by their very presence. Any other benefit conferred through this suppression, is coincidental. The purpose of allergy is not to expel helminths and is ineffective at doing so. There was another purpose for the allergic response.

In 2005, researchers suggested that the Toxin Hypothesis and the Helminth Hypothesis might fit together in a single causal framework. Allergic reactions intended to kill or expel parasites reduces their toxic effects the most serious of which is bladder cancer. The evolutionary reason for the allergic response may be in minimizing these carcinogenic hazards.[61]

Using the Helminth Hypothesis to explain the peanut allergy epidemic, however, was problematic. A study of children in Ghana, Africa with high levels of IgE to peanut and no clinical reactivity was explained by the suppressing "helminth effect".[62] This same effect, the cornerstone of the theory, does not apply in the US. 22 million Americans ostensibly free of major heminth infections were both sensitized and hyporeactive to peanut. This mass sensitization was identified by an ill publicized but no less significant US NHANE federal health survey.[63] The survey results of skin prick tests conducted between 1980 and 1994 were not published until 2001.

The absence of worms and the idea of a capricious Th2 drive to allergy did not explain the epidemiology of peanut allergy epidemic. It did not explain why primarily western toddlers were reacting, why just to peanut (or the other top 7 foods). And given that western countries have been largely unburdened by major helminth infections for decades, it did not explain the sudden accelerated prevalence of the allergy that began around 1990. Helminths in an investigation of peanut allergy appeared to be coincidental, not causal.

Hygiene Hypothesis

In 1989, British doctor David Strachan proposed a new explanation for the rise in hay fever, asthma and allergies. Observing that a decline in family size since the 1960s appeared to correlate with an increase in prevalence of allergy he speculated on how siblings affect the early development of the immune system. Strachan posited that infection and unhygienic contact with multiple siblings were important lessons for the young immune system. Reduced exposure to viral and bacterial pathogens that would otherwise have been brought home by older siblings and shared with younger ones had led to a skewed system that developed along Th2 rather than Th1 pathways, tending toward allergic conditions.

At the time, doctors were skeptical because most believed that infection was more of a trigger for allergy than a protection. However, the Hygiene Hypothesis grew in popularity and was supported by the example of Berlin. As already discussed, when the Berlin Wall came down in 1989, curious researchers found that in spite of lower levels of hygiene and vaccination and higher levels of pollution and smoking, East Germans rarely suffered from allergy or asthma. Within 10 years of reunification, however, allergy affected equal numbers on both sides of the city. Western children, it was then concluded, are too protected from infection by improvements in sanitation, chlorinated water, and medical interventions.[64] Adding to this sheltered existence was the reduced exposure to unhygienic siblings. Thus, the unnatural protections of a western lifestyle led to a rise in allergy. It seemed to fit.

In a 2000 article, Strachan re-iterated his belief in the protective power of infections that were "the most promising candidates" in staving off allergy.[65] The role of vaccination in the development of atopy, however, was dismissed because select studies on measles and pertussis had shown mixed results. As well, there seemed limited support for the possible roles of mycobacterial infection and overuse of antibiotics that reduced intestinal flora.

What stood out for Strachan 10 years after first proposing the theory were his original findings on variation of hay fever and allergy related to birth order – the tendency to atopy in the first birth and declining in youngest regardless of family size – and socioeconomic status. But these, he suggested, were clues to "the presence of a powerful underlying determinant of allergic sensitization". He suggested that the prevalence of hay fever and asthma was related to one's degree of exposure to this powerful and "true" protective factor.[66] The protective feature of this exposure also appeared to depend on timing.

And so, a renewed Hygiene Hypothesis in 2000 offered that insufficient exposure to an unknown infectious agent(s) that would afford a robust and balanced Th1-Th2 immune response and therefore protection from allergy was the cause of allergy. Others added the role of regulatory T cell responses (T reg) to this explanation.[67]

But just as the lack of pathogenic stimulation can create allergy so too can active viral and bacterial diseases that spread easily in crowded conditions of industrialized societies.[68] For example, researchers have correlated the onset of respiratory infections with onset of IgE mediated respiratory allergies in children. In one experiment, puppies injected at regular intervals with both pollen extracts and live viral vaccines mounted a significantly greater IgE response than did puppies injected only with pollen extracts.[69] The viruses or their toxic die off acted as adjuvants stimulating the production of IgE.

And while children in Ghana who have been exposed to siblings and have many illnesses also have many allergies. These children, however, are hyporeactive; they do not exhibit allergic symptoms to dust mites, for example, because they are "protected" by the immune suppressing effects of heavy parasitic infections.[70]

The Hygiene Hypothesis was touted as an explanation not just for asthma and hay fever they also for food allergy. Young in the *Peanut Allergy Answer Book* suggested that the absence of infections has "re-set" the immune system to target innocuous items in the child's diet resulting in "abnormal" reactions to peanut, for example.

In this explanation without a natural disease burden, the malfunctioning and capricious immune systems of children from too hygienic families have become little more than loose cannons. However, this view could not be reconciled with the basic facts of the peanut allergy epidemic – its sudden acceleration around 1990, in particular.

Nor did this hypothesis indicate a functional mechanism of mass sensitization to the peanut. How did these proteins access the blood streams of these children in different parts of the western world at the same time? It had already been established that consumption was irrelevant in the creation of these epidemic proportions; and that exposure through inhalation or skin cream was equally improbable.

The Hygiene Hypothesis did not offer a purpose for allergy. Given that severe allergy appears in all animals when specific proteins enter the blood stream, allergy would have an evolved purpose. As Margie Profet suggested, that purpose is a defense against toxins and any proteins associated with them.

In positing that homeostasis was impossible without a burden of disease, the Hygiene Hypothesis gave little credit to the human body. Evolutionary biologist Jared Diamond (b. 1937) pointed out that the thriving Native Americans had no infectious diseases to give back to the Europeans who landed in the Americas just 500 years ago.[71] The indigenous hunters and gatherers moved regularly thus preventing accumulation of toxins and pathogens from waste. Conversely,

European agricultural-based communities were sedentary. In living in close proximity with domestic animals and their wastes, Europeans and other farming societies infected themselves with viral and bacterial pathogens.

As Diamond pointed out, killer diseases are a legacy of 10,000 years of close contact with farm animals. Flu evolved from a disease of pigs transmitted via poultry. Measles was acquired from cattle; and smallpox, some believe, began in camels and moved to cattle. The Incas, unlike the Europeans, did not have the same history of close contact with domesticated animals. The Incas had llamas, but they were not milked, not kept in large herds, and they were not housed next to humans. According to Diamond, there was no significant exchange of germs between llamas and people.

Disease in humans grew from technological advance the consequences of which led to the creation of additional technologies – drugs, vaccines and antibiotics. In satisfying Strachan's observation that allergic sensitization was related to the timing and intensity of human exposure to a powerful underlying determinant, perhaps technology begged a closer look.

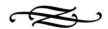

Part 2

A HISTORY OF MASS ALLERGY

Chapter 4

Re-discovering Anaphylaxis

Mass allergic phenomena emerged as a side effect of a late 19th century technology – vaccination.

Documented anaphylactic-like reactions prior to the 1890s were few and indeed the reaction itself appears to have been rare in history. A story of anaphylaxis was told in hieroglyphs regarding the reaction of Pharaoh Menes who died in 2640 BC from a wasp sting.[1] Hippocrates (460-375) described reactions to foods such as dairy that roused "a constituent of the body which is hostile to cheese". A fatality to a sting was reported by a French physician in 1765, thought to be the first documented case in Europe.

In the 19th century, French physiologist François Magendie (1783-1855) found that animals sensitized to egg white by injection went into shock and died after a subsequent injection.[2] Similar violent reactions in humans were believed to be rare "idiosyncrasies" that London doctor Jonathan Hutchinson (1828-1913) called "individuality run mad".[3] At the end of the 19th century, however, such reactions began to appear with startling frequency particularly in children. These reactions were produced following the application of a new technology, the hypodermic syringe to administer anti-toxin sera in the revolutionary treatment called vaccination.

Public tolerance of vaccination-induced allergy then simply called "serum sickness" was weighed against the fear of acquiring diseases in their natural form. Serum sickness was not fully understood until after 1901. At the dawn of the 20th century, immunologist and Nobel Laureate Charles Richet and pediatrician Clemens von Pirquet were able to show how the injection of vaccine proteins had caused the first allergy epidemic.

Justified behavior in the first lancet vaccination

Vaccination was developed in response to rampant and deadly infectious diseases in the western world. Many of these diseases in European and Asian societies had become a problem centuries ago when wastes from animal husbandry – the domestication of animals like cow, goat, pig, chicken and sheep – transferred viral and bacterial pathogens to humans. Unlike the hunter-gatherer societies, farming societies offered a more sedentary lifestyle in which just a few farmers could produce enough food for many people. Towns and villages grew up around the farms which flourished using plows, irrigation and manure fertilization. However, the inevitable run off of human and animal fecal matter with accompanying intestinal parasites and other contaminants drained into streams and rivers, infecting local sources of drinking water.

Again, as Jared Diamond pointed out, the Native American hunting and gathering societies did not have epidemic diseases to give back to the Europeans when they arrived in the New World.[4] Many indigenous populations like the Aztec and Incans in South America and the Huron and other tribes in North America were decimated by European smallpox and other deadly illnesses.

And arguably no less were Europeans devastated by their own diseases. Enhanced agricultural technologies in Europe meant that fewer people were required to work on farms. Without livelihood, uprooted populations crowded into larger industrialized communities looking for work. Densely populated cities like London or Paris that lacked proper waste disposal protocols until the mid to late 19th century encouraged the spread of disease; whether bubonic plague from the bite of infected fleas carried by rats or cholera from water contaminated with human feces.

These migrant peoples lured by the promise of land in North America also crowded onto ships. En route to their destinations, illness often swept through the close confines shared by hundreds of travellers. Once landed, health officials examined all arrivals and those who appeared ill were imprisoned in large quarantine tents.

Faced with a flood of immigrants and the threat of epidemic disease, officials required new laws and protocols for managing the waste and other problems that grew from crowding thousands of people into one small geographical area – London was the largest city in the world in 1900 with a population of about one million. This urbanizing trend also called "The Social Problem" forced many cities to formally incorporate and to develop departments of health to deal with bacteriology and disinfection.

Thus, the unnatural conditions of western progress – the shift from hunter-gatherer to agrarian and thence to industrial based societies – necessitated all manner of technical innovations not the least of which were in disease management. Fundamental to maintaining the health of westernized city populations were the sanitation of water systems, methods of waste disposal and the development of medicines and vaccines – which in turn seemed to produce new problems such as adverse reactions. Agriculture, Diamond re-iterated "was in many ways the greatest catastrophe from which we have never recovered."[5]

In the 18th century, smallpox also known as variola was a common and deadly disease that was often treated with infrequent success by variolation or inoculation. This technique named from the Latin inoculare (to graft) referred to the use of a lancet or sharp pronged tool to remove matter from a pustule of a smallpox victim and then to apply it under the skin – on the arm or leg – of a non-immune person. Any risk assumed from this crude treatment was more than justified when compared to acquiring the disease naturally at the time. There was a 20% to 60% chance of death from the terrifying natural form of smallpox acquired by two-thirds of the population of Western Europe in the mid-18th century. Well-justified fear easily dominated the conscious mind that was witness to so many agonizing deaths.

The worst strain of smallpox was blackpox. Blackpox caused the eyes to become dark red pits and the skin, darkened with hemorrhaging blood, to "slip off the body in sheets".[6] Ordinary smallpox caused the entire body, inside and out, to bubble up in painful infected blisters. When these pustules lost their pressure they leaked liters of the odorous pus until they finally crusted over in brown scabs. But the scabbing phase could be the most dangerous. Just as a victim seemed to have improved, it was common for the patient to suddenly bleed out internally oozing liquid from every orifice. Smallpox left the brain for last. Victims remained fully aware of their condition with their appetites intact until the end. Those who survived the disease were hideously scarred. And one third of these were left blind.[7]

Vaccination was initially developed to combat smallpox. When an outbreak occurred in Gloucestershire England in 1788, country doctor, Edward Jenner (1749-1823) observed that people, such as dairymaids, who worked with cattle, had much milder cases of the disease. Jenner deduced a connection between cowpox and smallpox and began to experiment with cow pus variolation. One of his first experiment volunteers was an eight-year-old boy. Jenner made wounds on the boy's skin and applied a liquid made from cowpox sores. After the patient's recovery from the milder cowpox, Jenner applied a smallpox liquid in the same manner. When the patient did not contract the disease Jenner was able to repeat his experiment on several children and adults. This time he used an arm-to-arm "passive" treatment, transferring pus from one person to another. Only four of these people were challenged by smallpox and found to be protected.

Jenner was subsequently lionized by the medical community as a hero whose experiments on children laid the foundation for disease management through childhood vaccination. Jenner's technique that he called "vaccination" in 1798 after the Latin word "vacca" for cow did have a precedent in at least one documented case in England. Farmer Benjamin Jesty (1737–1816) in the 1770s inoculated his own family using a darning needle and cow pus.

At his own expense, Jenner published his results – twelve experiments plus sixteen additional case histories he had collected since the 1770s – in the *Inquiry into the Causes and Effects of the Variolae Vaccine* (1798). This text was translated into a variety of languages including French, Italian and Dutch thereby introducing the vaccination technique to many countries.[8]

Jenner's work and the hope it engendered resulted in mass vaccination campaigns throughout Europe. By 1821, Denmark, Norway, Russia, Sweden and others had made infant vaccination compulsory. Vaccination was even taken to the Caribbean. In 1803, King Charles IV of Spain sent Francisco Xavier de Balmis to their colonies in the Americas on the "Royal Expedition of the Vaccine". Before leaving Spain, de Balmis kidnapped five Madrid orphans for the voyage. During the voyage, one child after the other was made ill with cowpox through arm-to-arm vaccination. In this way de Balmis kept the vaccine fresh until they arrived at their destination.[9]

Reflecting on the ethics of Jenner's experiments on children, one modern researcher stated that the doctor was justified given the devastating nature of smallpox at that time.[10] Jenner gambled his own life as well in this medical venture. The death of a child might have led to a charge of murder. And yet, patients embraced the cards of risk and reward dealt by the procedure. It was the lesser of two evils and if there were side effects, the patient gratefully assumed all responsibility for them.

It was soon discovered, however, that a single vaccination did not confer lifelong immunity. As well, inconsistent vaccination procedures used by doctors had actually led to the spread of cowpox and other diseases. Creative doctors would scratch or puncture the skin using a variety of unsanitary tools such as knives, forks, needles and pins in parallel, crosshatch, spiral, and geometric formations.[11] And the passive arm-to-arm vaccination method frequently transmitted secondary infections especially syphilis. Syphilis, called the Great Pox, was terrifying and fatal.

Under these conditions, the challenge of safe vaccine delivery seemed insuperable. A vaccine had to be created, transported and then administered. And it had to be done as safely as possible. Initially, an infected calf provided a fresh source of vaccine. The animal was led by foot or shipped from town to town where doctors or others would use the pus in the tradition of Jenner. Eventually, however, the calf would either recover or die thus ending the supply. In desperate times, cowpox scabs were packaged and mailed and then reconstituted. Finally, an antibacterial vegetable glycerin was added to liquid cowpox pus.[12] This mixture naturally decomposed within a short period of time prompting vaccine makers to include preservatives.

Despite the inconsistent results of Jenner's technology, it opened up the potential for managing other diseases in the same manner. The rapid speed with which vaccination and indeed technology of all kinds evolved during the 19th century was marked by impatience on the part of scientists.

Scientists Theodor Schwann and Mathias Schleiden in 1839 published the idea that plants and animals were made of cells, from the Latin "cellular" or room. It was a short step from cell biology to germ theory, a concept that marked the beginning of modern science based medicine. Louis Pasteur (1822-1895) refuted the idea that disease was spontaneously generated from ghost-like miasms. Disease was a manifestation of microorganisms in the environment or in the body. His German rival Koch used a microscope to identify in 1882 and 1883 respectively, the germs that caused tuberculosis and cholera.

And yet, the idea that invisible "germs" could make one sick was an astonishing idea. Even doctors had a hard time accepting the concept when it was first posited in a clinical setting. Hungarian physician Dr. Ignaz Semmelweis (1818-1865) in 1847 outraged his contemporaries by suggesting that just by washing their hands, doctors could save thousands of women from death in childbirth. Imprudently, Semmelweis persisted vociferously in his beliefs until his frightened wife believed he was losing his mind. In 1865, she had him committed to an asylum where he died two weeks later allegedly beaten to death by guards.

The public too resisted the idea that invisible germs were in the air, foods and water. In 1854, renowned public health worker John Snow had to convince London officials that an outbreak of cholera in Soho was being caused by a particular communal water well contaminated by human feces. Snow pioneered shoe-leather epidemiology, going door to door to trace the source of the outbreak. Finally, city officials removed the pump handle from a well on Broad Street thus ending the outbreak.

Such public breakthroughs gave doctors and men of science a new gloss of authority and social prestige – even the word "scientist" was new having just been coined in 1833 by English polymath William Whewell (1794-1866). Through the 19th century there emerged a parade of scientific innovations that produced both exciting and destabilizing effects. None of the technological advances was without problem or further opportunity.

An electric distribution system, patented in 1880 by Thomas Edison allowed him to capitalize on his invention of the electric lamp (one of his 1,093 US patents) spawning an explosion in electric devices. Scottish-born Alexander Graham Bell (1847-1922) patented the telephone in 1876 and engendered a communications revolution. German inventor and engineer Karl Benz (1844-1929) patented an internal combustion engine in 1879 for use in automobiles; he built the first horseless carriage, the patented Motorwagen, in 1885. The appeal of the automobile spurred the evolution of a massive petroleum industry (begun in 1846 with a method of refining it into kerosene).

Other 19th century inventions that had significance in daily life included the typewriter and the qwerty keyboard, the sewing machine, the toaster, the tin can (and the can opener) and, the invention that marked the entire century, mass production of all of these new devices.

Having no less an impact during this period of rapid industrialization and modernization was the rise of mass vaccination that grew from the success of Jenner and a long line of heroes in the study of immunology. On the heels of Jenner, Pasteur and Koch, scientists from France, Germany and England raced to develop vaccines – these countries funded and encouraged scientific advance because it enhanced their international profiles and because it led to improved technologies of war. These two goals seemed to come together in 1896 when the estate of Swedish inventor Alfred Nobel (1833-1896) revealed the multi-millionaire's will had established five prizes, three of which were for science.

Nobel who had made a fortune from his patented nitroglycerin dynamite was startled by the publication in 1888 of a premature obituary which called him a "merchant of death": "Dr. Alfred Nobel, who became rich by finding ways to kill more people faster than ever before died yesterday." From this, allegedly, Nobel was moved to create the $9 Million fund for the prizes as a more positive lasting legacy – especially in science.

The news of the Nobel prizes intensified the already heated competition between international vaccine scientists. In the first decade of the prizes, the majority of prizes in medicine went to those working on disease: the first Nobel Prize in Physiology and Medicine in 1901 went to Emil von Behring "for his work in serum therapy against diphtheria"; the 1902 prize went to Ronald Ross (UK, 1857-1932) "for his work on malaria"; in 1903 it was Niels Ryberg Finsen (Denmark, 1860-1904) for his work on lupus vulgaris and other diseases; 1905 to Robert Koch (Germany, 1843-1910) for his work in tuberculosis; 1907 to Charles Laveran (France, 1845-1922) for his understanding of protozoa in causing diseases; 1908 to Ilya Illyich Mechnikov (Russia, 1845-1916) and Paul Ehrlich (Germany, 1854-1915) for "their work on immunity".

Ingredients for a variety of vaccines evolved rapidly through the late 19th and early 20th centuries in order to extend vaccine shelf life and to make them more effective. Such ingredients eventually included a mercury based anti-fungal, oil excipients to enhance the reactivity of the body, carrier gels made from boiled animals, and more. Exact ingredients of these proprietary formulae held by commercial vaccine makers – and benefiting the scientists who developed them – were fiercely guarded by patent and corporate law, the cornerstone of which was shareholder protection. These protections and new legislation to protect the public from vaccine damage grew within an economic framework supported by the tradition of mass vaccination.

A framework for mass vaccination

Research and development in vaccines was aided by the invention of a new device making their administration easier and more effective, the hypodermic needle. At the same time, laying the framework for the production, distribution and sale of both vaccine and needle, were the business minded makers of patent medicines and pharmaceuticals. These proliferated in large numbers at the close of the US Civil War (1861-65).

The Civil War created an unprecedented demand for pharmaceuticals (from the Greek pharmakon or "remedy") including pain killers, anesthetics and smallpox vaccination materials. More soldiers on both Union and Confederate sides succumbed to disease than were killed in action. While an estimated 300,000 Union soldiers died during the war, only one third of these deaths were from war wounds. In deciding the outcome of the war, smallpox was a significant factor whether acquired naturally or deliberately through its use as a bio-weapon. There was at least one documented example of a Confederate doctor who knowingly sold smallpox-infected clothes to Union soldiers.[13]

Soldiers were expected to be vaccinated and they welcomed it. The vaccine medium consisted of glycerin and pulverized crusts or scabs from cowpox pustules obtained from vaccinated calves or children. However, late in the war, there was a shortage of all medicines including scabs. These, naturally, became valuable. Private physicians were paid $5. (about $70. in 2008) for each usable scab.[14] Some soldiers collected scabs and sent them home for their families to use and possibly sell. With drug shortages, blockade running or smuggling were methods by which doctors hoped to obtain these scabs and other drugs including quinine, chloroform, ether, opium, and morphine. In lieu of these, desperate doctors and druggists resorted to old remedy recipes using barks, leaves and roots of native plants. They used butterfly root for fever, red-oak bark and bicarbonate of soda as antiseptics, and poppy heads and nightshade to reduce pain.

Wartime lessons in creative drug innovation and the cost-effective mass manufacture of same had made business in pharmaceuticals potentially profitable. Aided by aggressive marketing and the expansion in the medicines industry north of the Mason-Dixon line, demand for cures of all kinds grew.

Many small companies sprang up at the close of the Civil War. Companies such as Upjohn (established in Michigan, 1885) made Heart Pills with nitroglycerin, digitalis, strophanthus and belladonna. The Eli Lilly Co., launched in 1876 by Civil War veteran and pharmacist Eli Lilly, produced cannibis tinctures, poisons, gelatin capsules for liquid medicines and Succus Alternas, a blood purifier for syphilis derived from a Creek Indian remedy.[15]

The late 19th century makers and sellers of patent or trademarked medicines on both sides of the Atlantic were dubbed "nostrum-mongers" by novelist Henry James – their products or *nostrum remedium* "our remedy" in Latin was shortened to "nostrum".

Patented nostrums that grew from 2,700 in 1880 to 38,000 by 1916 tended to have a high alcohol content and were fortified with morphine, opium or cocaine. Late 19th century remedies such as the German imported Bayer's powdered Heroin Hydorchloride intended to cure morphine addiction, Lloyd Brothers Cannabis in alcohol for gonorrhea, John Wyeth & Bros. Morphine and Chloroform cough syrup, or Mulford Co.'s Cotton-Root Bark abortion tincture were doubtless dangerous. These nostrums were sold using aggressive media campaigns that included print advertising, trademarks, lively packaging and promotional vehicles such as medical almanacs. The companies used saturation advertising and employed newspaper agents in the distribution of mail order products.[16]

Nostrum mongers frequently exaggerated the curative power of their remedies. Henry James's psychologist brother, William James, was so appalled by "the medical advertisement abomination" that in 1894 he declared that "the authors of these advertisements should be treated as public enemies and have no mercy shown".[17] And yet, many of these nostrum sellers in continuing to embrace advances in western medicine and science grew into profitable modern pharmaceutical companies.

Parke-Davis (est. 1866, Detroit) that began in the sale of herbal remedies became the largest US pharmaceutical company with annual sales of more than $3 Million in the 1890s – the rough equivalent in 2008 of $73 Million. This company dominated the vaccine market that grew quickly beyond just smallpox. Next to "Modified Mixed Infection" vaccines – with License No. 1 issued in 1902 by the Secretary of the Treasury U.S.A. – the company sold such remedies as cocaine tablets to cure morphine addiction and buttermilk pills for invalids.

In the nostrum monger tradition, Parke-Davis founded medical publications such as the influential *Therapeutic Gazette* (published by company co-owner George S. Davis)[18] and supported others such as the *Index Medicus*, an index guide to medical journal articles catalogued initially by US Army doctor and book lover John Shaw Billings (1838-1913). Parke Davis also collaborated with members of the academic medical community, recruiting some for its research labs as it did in 1895 when it hired E.M. Houghton from the University of Michigan. By the 1890s, companies were able to hire workers trained in bacteriology, which was for the first time offered in medical school curricula.

As the US economy expanded, pharmaceutical companies enlarged both their manufacturing operations and their sales forces so that they were able to reach the doctors who were servicing fast-growing urban populations across the country.

The marketing methods for vaccines and anti-toxins in the 1890s resembled that used for pharmaceuticals today. Pharma company sales reps visited physicians to market the products, and left promotional sales literature including reprints of medical articles. One pamphlet quoted diphtheria fatality rates of 34.8% to 62.5% without anti-toxin, but 4.6% to 17.6% with it.[19] Parke-Davis competitor Mulford Co. was aggressive in its sales literature for diphtheria anti-toxin telling doctors: "Don't be afraid to use the anti-toxin. Don't be afraid of a large dose. Don't wait for result of a culture before use." Similarly, an 1897 Parke-Davis advertisement proclaimed: "We have never yet had reported a case of sudden death following the use of our Anti-toxin."[20]

However, by 1901-1902 there were several deaths related to the commercially produced smallpox and diphtheria vaccines.

Diphtheria, dubbed the 'strangling angel', is a bacterial infection that causes the lymph glands, throat and neck to swell. In severe cases the patient can suffocate. A milder form of diphtheria can also create skin lesions. Between 1891-1900 in London, there were 2.98 deaths from diphtheria per 1,000 children under age 5; between 1891-94 there were 548 deaths in the city. This rate was lower outside the major cities.[21]

In the 1890s, the German physician Emil von Behring developed an "anti-toxic" or protective serum that did not kill the diphtheria bacterium, but rather helped neutralize the toxic poisons that the bacterium released into the body. Von Behring created the anti-toxin from the blood (serum) of patients infected with diphtheria and from vaccinated animals. Von Behring first successfully used his anti-toxin serum on a child with the disease in 1891. His vaccine was likely the single most important catalyst in the creation of the science based pharmaceutical industry.[22] It brought him considerable wealth and fame.

Mass production and administration of the anti-toxin sera followed this success. Commercial and government laboratories used blood from farm animals in order to meet the enormous demand for the vaccine.[23] Horses were thought ideal animals in which to produce anti-toxin because they were large and highly reactive to diphtheria. A report in the NY Times told the story of one horse worth $175,000 to the City of New York.[24] Used by the Street Cleaning Dept., Horse 397 was ready for the glue factor when an enterprising doctor recruited him for the NY Health Department's Otisville laboratories (established in 1894). The horse was infected with diphtheria and bled twice a week producing 232,800,000 units of anti-toxin over two years.

The mass vaccination of children with such anti-toxin sera resulted in an apparent reduction in mortality rates. More than 30 articles heralded this outcome in the popular press in the US in 1894 and 1895.

Despite the success, however, injections were well known to cause a poorly understood and potentially fatal illness known at this time as "serum sickness".

Lab animals and horses repeatedly immunized with tetanus or diphtheria antigens to produce the antisera were often afflicted with serum sickness. Horses were known to suddenly collapse and die after a second or third injection. In humans, the condition made headlines after the daughter of renowned pathologist Paul Langerhans died within minutes of a diphtheria antiserum injection. In fact, serum sickness ravaged thousands of children causing fevers, rash, diarrhea, falling blood pressure, joint pain, breathing difficulties and other symptoms.

Diphtheria serum deaths soon made headlines in Norway, Hungary in 1895 and in the US in 1901.[25]

In 1901, a five-year-old child was admitted to a St. Louis hospital for treatment of a diphtheria infection. She received two anti-toxin shots. Nine days later, she died from tetanus. An ensuing investigation revealed that the Health Dept. for the City of St. Louis had produced diphtheria anti-toxin using a horse that had died of tetanus – the horse had been used to produce in excess of 30 quarts of anti-toxin over a three-year period. Two flasks of serum from the deceased horse were reportedly dumped down a laboratory sink. In reality, it was shown that the batch had actually been distributed to physicians. An additional 12 children died from tetanus shortly after the first. Another 100 cases of post-vaccinal tetanus occurred in New Jersey in 1901 with nine fatalities. The media called these children "anti-toxin victims".[26]

A standard for diphtheria anti-toxin had been developed in 1895, by the Hygienic Laboratory, an arm of the U.S. Marine Hospital Service. The Lab was later renamed the Public Health Service. While the government produced vaccines along side corporate enterprises at this time, the Hygienic Laboratory officials warned of "what will evidently ensue in our country. Many persons will commence to prepare the (antidiphtheria) serum as a business enterprise, and there will, without a doubt, be many worthless articles called anti-toxin thrown upon the market. All the serum intended for sale should be made or tested by competent persons."[27]

Government's role in building the tradition of vaccination gradually shifted from production to purely regulatory and administrative. Regulatory intervention began with the 1902 Biologics Control Act making the Hygienic Laboratory responsible for issuing licenses to makers of biologics that included vaccines – 13 businesses were licensed in 1904. This number grew quickly from 24 businesses in 1908 to 41 in 1921 producing over 100 biologics.[28]

But safety was not the only vaccine related concern of government. In 1906, a charge of conspiracy in price fixing was brought against the "Drug Trust of the United States". The Proprietary Association (for holders of patent medicines) and the Wholesale and Retail Druggists Associations as well as certain individuals were charged with violating Sherman Anti-trust laws.[29] In addition, there were long held concerns regarding false and misleading nostrum advertising that reporter Samuel Adams (1871-1958) called "The Great American Fraud" in *Collier's Weekly* (1905). The Pure Food and Drug Act passed in 1906 attempted to control false claims related to ingredients. These government actions helped restore public confidence in vaccination.

Despite the apparent acrimonious relationship, the lawsuits and tightening controls that continued with a 1936 ban on use of certain ingredients such as alcohol and narcotics, government needed pharmaceutical companies and their vaccines. Vaccination, its easy administration and promise of better odds against disease, was logically tied to the government's bottom line, economic growth. A sick population spelled the financial decline of a city or even a country. And they knew from bitter lessons learned during the US Civil War, that a disease afflicted army could lose.

The tradition of compulsory injections for US soldiers began in World War I (1914-1918) with vaccines for typhoid, cholera, tetanus, smallpox and other diseases. For the nostrum mongers that had grown into lucrative science-based pharmaceutical companies, government was a valuable customer that could and would influence and even enforce the buying decisions of the public. This see-saw relationship was woven into a complex fabric of conflicting concerns and desires that included the reputations and incomes of doctors and scientists, the interests of powerful medical associations, shareholders, the authority of government and the media which in its turn was supported by rich ad sales from pharmaceutical companies. The net result was a pattern of increasing drug and vaccine consumption in western industrialized countries that transformed the patient into a medical consumer.[30]

The neglected role of the needle

Medical consumers gradually embraced the tradition of vaccination by injection. Any concerns they had about the treatment focused naturally on reactions to the vaccine ingredients – the "anti-toxin" victims a case in point. In the creation of these poorly understood adverse reactions, however, few seemed aware of the significant role and meaning of the device that had made modern vaccination possible, the hypodermic needle.

The syringe with a needle fine enough to pierce the skin was developed independently in 1853 by Frenchman physician Charles Pravaz (1791-1853) and Scottish physician Alexander Wood (1817-1884). It was Wood, however, who in 1858 first publicized his "hypodermic" or beneath the skin needle as an ideal method for introducing morphine directly into the bloodstream. Wood's paper "A new method of treating neuralgia by the direct application of opiates to the painful points" in the *Edinburgh Medical and Surgical Review*, reported excellent results. The needle, which made the effect of morphine, a principal ingredient of opium,[31] at once immediate and more powerful than ingestion of same, was rapidly embraced by doctors and by the public in Europe and America. Florence Nightingale (1820-1910) pioneering nurse of the Crimean War (1853-56) wrote during her later years of illness, "Nothing did me any good, but a curious little new fangled operation of putting opium under the skin which relieved one for twenty-four hours."

The convenience and enhanced potency offered by this direct introduction to the bloodstream contributed to the increased prevalence of opiate addiction. Injected morphine used by doctors to treat the wounded during the US Civil War resulted in an alleged post-war malady called Soldier's Disease – in effect, thousands of veterans were made addicts. While this assertion has been debated, it remains a fact that the needle led to a rise in the medical and non-medical demand for morphine and its derivatives. One derivative was heroin, which was brought to market by Bayer in 1898. Morphine addiction was also the ultimate outcome for the hypodermic inventor Wood as well as his wife. Her eventual overdose is believed to be the first such recorded death.

The first to use the hypodermic needle to inject a vaccine was Louis Pasteur. His initial use of the device in the development of his anthrax vaccine for livestock[32] was followed in 1885 by vaccination of a young boy who had been bitten by a rabid dog.[33] Until Pasteur, vaccination referred only to cowpox and smallpox. Pasteur redefined vaccine as a live or inactivated microorganisms (bacteria, viruses) injected in order to induce immunity and to help prevent infectious disease.

Gradually, the hypodermic needle began to replace the unsteady and messy transdermal tools that were used to puncture or scratch the skin. There were few obstacles to the widespread use of the needle for vaccination. The cost was reasonable at $2.50 per device in 1897 (about $67. in 2008). Improvements on the design were required – the glass barrels tended to crack, tips leaked and needles easily snapped.

Production of liquid vaccines suited to the features of the hypodermic needle quickly followed. Vaccines in vegetable glycerin were developed for scarlet fever, yellow fever, snakebite, tuberculosis and more by the end of the century. Vaccines were mass-produced, packaged in vials, stored and shipped doctors in distant places. The needle made the mass administration of vaccines convenient, cost effective and relatively sanitary; the re-useable metal needles could be boiled or dipped in alcohol to kill bacteria. The graduated scale on the side of the glass barrel meant that serum could be measured. This was especially important given the noticeably stronger and immediate effects of injection.

Oral administration of drugs reduced and slowed their effects because of the natural action of digestive enzymes that destroyed and eliminated them. Injection seemed to be a better method of administration because it made the drug more potent. In the application of vaccines, however, bypassing the digestive system would prove to be far more problematic.

The convenient packaging of the needle with anti-toxin starting in the 1890s had wholly unforeseen outcomes. The shot pried the lid off a Pandora's box and unwittingly exposed those vaccinated to a host of man-made chronic degenerative diseases. The first was the life threatening allergic condition known as serum sickness. While vaccine innovation reduced the prevalence of serum sickness as the century unfolded (horses and sheep as sources for anti-toxin were replaced by lab samples such as chicken embryos and small animals) this episode in the history of vaccination provided an open window onto the ease with which allergic conditions can be created by the expedient of injection.

Serum sickness: the first man-made mass allergic phenomenon

Serum sickness was a condition that included the then yet-to-be-named anaphylaxis. The sickness was a common outcome of the first mass injections of anti-toxin sera for scarlet fever, tetanus and diphtheria before the turn of the century. Symptoms of serum sickness ranged from rashes, joint pain, fever, lymph node swelling, decreased blood pressure, enlarged spleen, kidney failure, breathing difficulty and shock which sometimes killed the patient.[34][35]

With the mass administration of injected sera, sickness occurred according to one writer in 1941 about "once in every seven hundred treatments" in the early decades of the 20th century.[36] Another writer put that number much higher with a 10% chance of developing acute serum sickness.[37] Yet another in 1934 believed it to be 50%.[38] The immediate effects of post-vaccinal serum sickness could last days, weeks, months or might never clear, leaving the victim in a chronic state of ill health and reactive to a range of substances including the vaccines themselves.

Austrian pediatrician Clemens Von Pirquet (1874-1929) and his Hungarian colleague, Béla Schick (1877-1967) studied serum sickness in thousands of children subjected to injections of antitoxic sera. In his detailed examinations of the children at the Universitats Kinderklinik in Vienna, Von Pirquet showed that the diverse manifestations of serum sickness were similar to those noted in hypersensitive reactions to strawberries, crabs, pollens and the poisons of bees and mosquitoes.

Von Pirquet postulated a close and seemingly paradoxical relationship between the two outcomes of vaccination: the process of becoming immunized and the hypersensitive characteristics of serum sickness. In both cases there was an incubation period between initial injection and appearance of symptoms; subsequent injections (like secondary exposure to infection) were accompanied by accelerated and exaggerated responses resulting from "a collision of antigen and antibody".[39]

There were, he also noted, idiosyncrasies or individual variations in response to sera related to dose and injection intervals. Immediate adverse reaction in 90% of his patients had occurred following the second injections 10 to 30 days after the first. Von Pirquet concluded that the length of incubation time depended not only upon the foreign body or antigen but also upon the organism in question, the person.[40] Finally in 1906, he reconciled the two outcomes of vaccination – immunity and hypersensitivity – in a new framework of altered reactivity he called "allergy".[41]   The modern concept of allergy grew from the study of the vaccination provoked mass allergy, serum sickness.

The prevalence of serum sickness posed a dilemma for authorities, doctors and government. Warren Vaughan summarized this concern in *Strange Malady* (1941):

> Serum disease, as this is called, is a man-
> made malady. If we had no curative serums
> and if there were no such thing as a
> hypodermic syringe with which to introduce
> the material under the skin, there would be
> no serum disease. Instead multitudes would
> still be dying from diphtheria and lockjaw
> and several other infections. Thus we find
> ourselves in somewhat of a dilemma, faced
> with the necessity for choosing the lesser of
> two potential evils. [42]

In England, there was no legal choice between the two "evils" until 1898. In the US, mandatory vaccination laws – that included quarantine and isolation – were primarily the responsibility of state and local governments. In 1827, Boston was the first city to require smallpox vaccination for public school students. Other cities and states followed with their own mandatory vaccination laws. Legislation developed based on changes in disease and available vaccines.

But the British public was uneasy about vaccination and there were levels of non-compliance with the compulsory law – some preferred to take their chances with the disease.

Throughout much of the 19ᵗʰ century, the passive arm-to-arm technique for smallpox was used at the vaccination stations around England. Paid "vaccinators" would apply matter to multiple sites on the arms, legs of children. Since the vaccinators received a commission for every certificate of successful vaccination they were motivated to treat as many people as possible. Aggressive vaccinators were loathed by many mothers who were fearful of the often contaminated matter and yet were forced by law to submit their children to the treatment.[43] Mothers who refused vaccination were hunted and found. Also known as "baby hunters", the government vaccinators used entrapment techniques to unearth dodgers. Parents with means, on the other hand, paid for calf lymph and the services of a doctor.[44]

As the lancet made way for the syringe, severe criticism of the perceived panacea of vaccination came from the public and some doctors in Europe and the US. It was suggested that vaccination might actually have spread smallpox. In *Vaccine Delusion* (1898) British naturalist Alfred Wallace questioned the efficacy of vaccination. He used statistics and charts to prove that smallpox increased significantly with the administration of vaccination.

Others believed that the disease had declined as a result of improved sanitation (bed bugs were believed to carry the disease) and waste disposal protocols and natural nutrition led by health crusaders such as Sylvester Graham (1795-1851).[45] [46] Graham was a Presbyterian minister and vegetarian who created not only a system of living but also healthful foods such as the Graham cracker.

Dr. William Young in *Killed by Vaccination* (1887) objected to the "useless, cruel and inhuman law of compulsory vaccination under cover of which, as has been stated in the House of Commons, children are slaughtered by wholesale."

Socialist playwright George Bernard Shaw (1856-1950) joined the opposition to smallpox vaccination in spite of having nearly died from the disease in 1881. In the 1909 Preface to *The Doctor's Dilemma* (1906) he expounded on the perils of vaccination. He cited the example of Koch's 1894 tuberculin vaccine the results of which "…were not accidents, but perfectly orderly and inevitable phenomena following the injection of dangerously strong 'vaccines' at the wrong moment, and reinforcing the disease instead of stimulating the resistance to it."[47]

Shaw pointed to the process of opsonization in which an antigen is marked for destruction by a phagocyte. Antibodies, for example, will coat an antigen. The antibodies then bind to receptors on the membrane of the phagocytic cells that in turn ingest the antigen. This, Shaw suggested, was a concept well beyond the understanding of most doctors. Not only did doctors not understand the risks of vaccination, argued Shaw, but also they were in it for the money. Vaccines were cheap to make and lucrative in their application.

And an epidemic "windfall" made the job of vaccinators and doctors even more lucrative, opined Shaw. An outbreak inspired a panic and rush for vaccination, which would then be "defended desperately were it twice as dirty, dangerous and unscientific than it is". Vaccination is not about science, it's about economics, declared Shaw.

In 1898, the British government switched to calf lymph suspended in glycerin for a still disconcerted public stating that this new vaccine was purified. This improvement was perhaps a concession that paved the way for a new vaccination technique using the hypodermic syringe. The needle, however, was not much of an advance for mothers of children who began to exhibit a host of strange, new reactions after injection.

Serum sickness to the injected vaccine was unlike anything provoked by the vaccinator's contaminated cowpox pus. It was the first man-made allergic phenomenon created en mass in children.

Discovery of food anaphylaxis

It was during his famous 1901 vaccination experiments on dogs that French immunologist Charles Richet (1850-1935) discovered what he termed anaphylaxis.

Richet and his colleague Paul Portier were onboard the yacht of oceanographer Prince Albert I of Monaco to explore the possibly of producing a vaccine to physalia poison, a toxin from the tentacles of the Portuguese Man of War. The scientists began by injecting dogs with the toxin. Dogs that survived were given time to recover and then re-injected.

Richet expected that the first exposure to the poison would have created a certain amount of immunity in the dogs. Instead, the initial exposure made the dogs hypersensitive. A second, much smaller dose of toxin caused a violent reaction akin to serum sickness that quickly killed them. In his lab, Richet soon discovered that even a small dose of proteins injected into a dog followed by another small dose several weeks later produced the same result.

This deadly reaction, Richet observed, depended not upon the dose (contrary to von Pirquet) since even the smallest dose would trigger it, but upon the time interval between injections (similar to von Pirquet). Further research by Nicolas Arthus in 1903 and Richard Otto in 1905 showed that without exception all proteins toxic or non-toxic could produce anaphylaxis through injection – egg, milk, meat, diphtheria. And although the key again was interval, this incubation period also varied between species and between substances.

To describe this phenomenon, Richet paired two Greek words in anaphylaxis – "ana" against and "phylaxis" protection – essentially the opposite outcome they sought with vaccination.[18] In his acceptance speech for the 1913 Nobel Prize in Medicine, Richet described anaphylaxis as one of three possible outcomes of vaccination. These were: unchanged sensitivity or stability; diminished sensitivity or habituation; and heightened sensitivity. The first injection, instead of protecting the organism, wrote Richet, rendered it more fragile and susceptible. After an incubation period of several weeks, a second injection of the same proteins triggered anaphylaxis.[49]

Alimentary or food anaphylaxis, Richet had discovered through experiments, was the body's defensive response to proteins that had by-passed the modifying process of the digestive system and been introduced directly to the blood stream.[50]

By injection, Richet sensitized dogs, cats, rabbits, horses and frogs to a variety of foods showing that the phenomenon is universal to all animals. For example, he created anaphylaxis to raw meat in dogs. Initially, he fed the animals cooked meat and measured their leucocyte or white blood cell levels that were normal. When he fed the dogs raw meat, white blood cell levels quickly increased. Richet deduced from this that "digestive juices" were required to modify the proteins of the raw meat and if this was not accomplished the body would mount an immune response. Subsequently, Richet injected raw meat proteins into the dogs which provoked an anaphylactic reaction.[51]

Dogs, of course, eat raw meat all the time without developing anaphylaxis. At a 1913 International Medical Congress in London, Richet confirmed that it was difficult to bring about food anaphylaxis by just eating a food:

> Experimental alimentary anaphylaxis is
> difficult to bring about under conditions of
> healthy digestion, since it is a question of
> toxalbumins or nutritive albumins...
> because the digestive juices actively
> intervene in transforming these albumins
> and rendering them innocuous...[52]

Another aspect to anaphylaxis was specificity in identity between the preparatory and unleashing substances. Richet identified the phenomena of cross reactivity of "allied protein groups" when he found that the injection of milk from different animals produced similar anaphylactic symptoms in a sensitized dog.

Significantly, Richet also observed that the incubation period between sensitizing and unleashing injections varied according to the substance used. A minimum period of one week between injections was indicated to create anaphylaxis to milk in a guinea pig but two weeks for mussel protein.[53]

Despite his view that anaphylaxis was universal, all animals were subject to it, Richet had little sympathy for those who acquired it through vaccination. In fact, a highly prejudicial concept of biological superiority and evolutionary socialism informed Richet's view of anaphylaxis related to vaccination. Post-vaccinal anaphylaxis weeded out the weak:

> Anaphylaxis is thus necessary to the
> species, often to the detriment of the
> individual. The individual may perish, but
> this does not matter. The species must at
> all times retain its organic integrity.

Anaphylaxis defends the species against
the peril of adulteration.[54]

The origins of the Ingestion Hypothesis

Although anaphylactic reactions to sera were common among children, food anaphylaxis in a clinical setting was not. And because it was uncommon, there was a struggle to provide an in-the-field explanation for its rare appearance. Literature reveals that doctors began to dismantle and boil down the landmark observations of Richet, to pick and choose bits that seemed to provide that explanation.

Doctors relied on one aspect of Richet's anaphylaxis research. Richet had stated that food sensitization occurred when proteins unmodified by the digestive system entered the blood stream. And so, ingestion of food by persons with inadequate digestion appeared to be a common sense prerequisite for food allergy. It was an idea that explained the increasing caseload of non-life threatening food allergies, and it seemed to fit those rare cases of food anaphylaxis. At the time, these reactions were primarily to egg, but also to fish and dairy.[55]

Of the two "how to" mechanisms Richet had employed in his experiments, ingestion and injection, the latter was exorcised from the nascent Ingestion Hypothesis. It was assumed that children with food anaphylaxis had unhealthy digestion. There was little interest in other physical conditions that might contribute to individual sensitization. In fact, observed differences between animals in anaphylaxis experiments constituted "noise" rather than a signal to researchers.[56]

Not that food anaphylaxis was impossible to produce through ingestion alone. A problem, yet unidentified, was that this cursory and incomplete theory became a knee jerk explanation even as food anaphylaxis increased through the decades. At the time, however, demand for more research on the problem was limited. Food anaphylaxis was rare.

A rare case of "egg poisoning", in which a boy suffered from angioedema and asthma after eating the food, was reported in 1908 by English physician Alfred Schofield.[57] Another in 1912 was described as an idiosyncrasy by a New York pediatrician, Oscar Schloss. A child at 10 days of age was given raw egg white to calm diarrhea. He next ate egg at 14 months of age at which time "he cried out, clawed at his mouth, and his tongue and mouth swelled until they were many times normal size." Schloss suggested that the boy's experience might be due to a new condition that had been receiving so much attention, called allergy.

To confirm his suspicions, Schloss injected the boy's blood into a guinea pig. Later he injected egg white. The animal went into anaphylactic shock.[58]

To prove anaphylaxis, doctors used injection – a dramatic and arguably unnecessary gesture. And yet, as a mechanism that might explain the boy's initial sensitization the needle was simply not considered.

Another rare anaphylactic reaction was reported in "Absorption of Undigested Protein from the Alimentary Tract as Determined by the Direct Anaphylaxis Test"[59] in the *America Journal of Physiology* in 1925. The de facto conclusion in the title of the article revealed how entrenched the Ingestion Hypothesis had become. Vaccination as a mechanism of sensitization was not considered even as the authors of the article unleashed food anaphylaxis by injecting yet another guinea pig with blood from the egg allergic patient. An "intoxicating dose of the suspected protein (egg white) was injected intraperitoneally into the test animal resulting in anaphylaxis." The authors did not pose the question that from today's perspective would be most salient, why egg? Why not peanut, for example?

The expeditious Ingestion Hypothesis was handed down through 20th century medical literature because it explained the vast majority of food reactions. These reactions manifested not in anaphylaxis but in a variety of uncomfortable and hard to diagnose symptoms such as migraines, digestive upsets, skin conditions, fatigue, anxiety, irritability and behavioral problems.[60] As early as 1905, Dr. Francis Hare had written *The Food Factor in Disease*, a two volume book that recommended elimination diets to help manage disease. The relationship of food sensitivity and disease appeared sporadically in medical journals such as the *Archives of Internal Medicine, Journal of the American Medical Association, and Annals of Clinical Medicine* in the 1920s and onward.[61] The editorial for the first 1929 issue of the US *Journal of Allergy* explained that the clinical use of the word allergy was to describe a broad variety of symptoms to as many substances. Anaphylaxis was reserved for those rare and violent reactions.

Vaughan's *Strange Malady* summarized the thinking about food anaphylaxis at the time. Vaughan again explained the Ingestion Hypothesis related to intestinal permeability that resulted in the escape of proteins into the blood stream:

> How can one become allergic to egg when nobody has ever injected egg into him? Under certain conditions egg protein taken by mouth may be absorbed undigested through the intestines and into the blood just as though it had been injected through the skin. A period of indigestion, some vitamin deficiency favoring abnormal absorption, overeating, temporary

> disturbance in the activity of the digestive
> juices or some other factor might promote
> absorption of undigested protein.[62]

Vaughan assumed that egg had never been injected – and he may have been correct but the fact was that injection was rejected outright as even a possible mechanism of sensitization.

And yet, emulsified egg lecithin had been used extensively in vaccines prior to the publication of Vaughan's book. In 1931, vaccine manufacturers had introduced fertile hen's egg as a medium for growing viruses. This was seen as an advance because vaccines grown on mouse brain had produced allergic brain encephalitis in some children.[63] Vaughan, however, stated that adverse vaccine reactions including the man-made serum sickness had all but vanished in 1941 due to the improvements in "purifying serums".[64]

In one sentence the doctor removed vaccination from the discussion of anaphylaxis altogether. He was satisfied to focus on consumption as the cause of sensitization even in babies in utero. He pointed to mothers whose "abnormal food cravings" during pregnancy might cause of sensitization. The doctor did not see the problem in his logic when he stated that food anaphylaxis is an "abnormal" reaction *primarily* to egg. If anaphylaxis was almost always to egg, how could it be abnormal?

Something linked the egg allergic patients. Again, why egg and not beef or pork or any of the thousands of proteins children and mothers ate at this time including peanuts, an inexpensive staple in US households?

Peanut allergy was unknown at this time. Vaughan mentioned peanuts once in his book but as a crushed topping and nothing more. Among the foods to which people had developed allergies, peanut appeared not to be one of them.

Even in the course of attempting to reverse anaphylaxis through "anti-anaphylaxis" injection treatments, the mechanism of injection was never implicated in the creation of anaphylaxis related to food.

Like trying to put the genie back in the bottle, early allergists used repeated "sub-anaphylactic" doses of substances to de-sensitize allergy sufferers. Jay Schamberg had observed in 1919 that tolerance to poison ivy in Native American populations was achieved through the preventive practice of chewing poison ivy shoots. Richard Otto contended that the anaphylactic antibody might become exhausted or neutralized by injections of the substances to which one was allergic. However, these injections proved to be a temporary reprieve for most and tended to provoke anaphylactic reactions. [65]

And so, the incomplete Ingestion Hypothesis persisted as a blanket explanation for food anaphylaxis. And it remained so even during the first outbreak of food anaphylaxis that occurred to one food starting in the late 1930s. Literature revealed a sudden surge in anaphylaxis to cottonseed oil in the US that peaked in the 1940s and dissipated through the 50s.

The first outbreak of food anaphylaxis

Research in clinical allergy grew slowly and not at all in anaphylaxis. Infectious disease continued to dominate the attention of doctors and pharmaceutical companies. Great strides were made during WW II in the development of injected antibiotics. This "wonder drug" developed in 1928 by Scottish-born biologist Alexander Fleming (1881-1955) promised cures for all manner of infections from gonorrhea to tonsillitis. But it was during the war for treatment of wounded soldiers that solutions were found to mass production of the drug.

In 1942, the Pfizer Company in Brooklyn, NY emerged as the leader in mass production of penicillin because of its historical expertise in fermentation. By 1944, this and other companies had met the demand for the injected drug that included a homegrown oil excipient, refined cottonseed oil.[66] [67]

Before WW II, experiments with food oil excipients in vaccines included oil from castor bean, cottonseed, corn, olives and more. Starting as early as 1913, these oils were often emulsified with hydrolyzed casein (dairy protein) or egg lecithin.[68] An emulsion is a mixture of two or more immiscible liquids. One liquid is dispersed in another; the most common being oil and water into which a surface active substance can increase the stability of the mixture so that it can be stored for lengthy periods.

Yanol produced in Japan, for example, was an emulsion made from 3% castoreum (oil secreted by beavers) and stabilized by egg lecithin. Tested in the US in the 1930s this product had to be withdrawn due to side effects such as shaking fits, fever and anaphylaxis. In the 1940s a second generation of fat emulsions emerged. The best known on the market under the name Lipomul introduced in 1935 and marketed in the 40s was made with refined cottonseed oil.

The process of refining the oil for use in these excipients was crucial. This process removed proteins from the oil, well known by this time to cause allergic sensitization if injected. As it was, many side effects occurred with this oil such as vomiting, shaking fits, tachycardia, drop in blood pressure, difficulties breathing and shock.[69] Cottonseed oil contains the toxic steroid gossypol which became a common agricultural pesticide.

Concerns regarding the "anaphylactogenic potency" of cottonseed emerged before 1943.[70] Warren Vaughan warned cottonseed allergic readers to be aware of this hidden ingredient in many processed foods including mayonnaise, vegetable shortening, canned tuna.[71] Sensitivity to cottonseed oil grew through the 1930s and was still a concern in 1950.[72] [73]

In 1947, worries over the spread of cottonseed allergy and increasing allergic reactions to processed foods were taken to a committee at the US Federal Security Agency. Testimony given before the Agency was published in a 1949 report.

At the inquiry, two out of six doctors challenged the assertion that refined cottonseed oil was actually free from allergenic proteins.[74] Testimony from oil processing technicians revealed that the machinery used for the commercial refining of cottonseed oil was not thoroughly cleaned before it was used for the refining of another oil. These sloppy procedures, it was suggested, had led to the contamination of various oils with cottonseed oil.[75] It was suggested that this hidden contaminant had resulted in an outbreak of anaphylactic reactions. None though, ventured to inquire into the causes of initial sensitization.

While the Association of Cottonseed Products argued that food labels did not need to list the refined oil because it was free of allergens, suspicion remained regarding the quality of cottonseed oil.

An explanation for the inconsistency in the quality of the oil and the resulting cross contamination may have begun with a challenged cottonseed industry weakened by bad deals, bad luck and the Depression. Between 1909 and 1920 a boll weevil blight saw the price of cotton tumble from 34.98 cents per pound in 1919 to 9.4 cents per pound, causing the agricultural crisis of 1920-21. The Crash of 1929 and drought from 1929-39 forced many cotton farmers from the land. The number of cotton farms fell from 123,477 to 86,889 in Oklahoma alone and harvested acreage decreased dramatically from over 4 million to 1.6 million. Declining production marked the industry for the remainder of the 20th century.[76]

Adding to this misery was a conflict over seed grading between the Cottonseed Crushers' Association and the federal government, the USDA. In 1930-31, attempts to come to an agreement were stalled when a Federal Trade Commission found rule violations. In addition, 1930s New Deal acreage allotments reduced cottonseed yields. As a result of these challenges, the availability of cottonseed oil began to diminish.

By the late 40s, cottonseed oil was demoted to minor product in the competitive food oils industry[77] and it was largely but not entirely replaced in the delivery of vaccines and drugs. At the same time, the prevalence of cottonseed anaphylaxis fell. Intense interest in this allergy in the 1940s dropped sharply through the 1950s. Infrequent titles appear subsequently in the medical literature with an unusual report of its re-emergence in the 1980s.[78]

In choosing a vegetable oil replacement for the unreliable cottonseed oil, US vaccine makers chose one that was tariff protected, cheap, abundant, and home-grown – its availability had made it an important source of glycerin in the manufacture of explosives during the two World Wars.

After WW II, the all American peanut replaced cottonseed as the oil ingredient of choice in the manufacture of penicillin and vaccines.[79]

Chapter 5

A History of Peanut Allergy

Peanut oil in penicillin

In Queens, New York during the summer of 1943, two-year-old Patricia Malone was dying. She had been diagnosed with acute staphlococcic septicemia, a bacteria that had left her delirious, and barely breathing. On August 15th at twenty to four in the afternoon the city editor of the *New York Journal –American* received a call from the child's father. She had only seven hours to live unless she received the new drug called penicillin.

Penicillin was difficult to obtain and make in large quantities. It took a chemist a whole day to produce just one small flask of it. And even then, one dose of the "wonder drug" would last for just three hours before being excreted by the kidneys. Worse yet, penicillin was under severe restrictions during the war. The only man authorized to release the antibiotic to civilians was Dr. Chester Keffer in Boston. Through a series of frantic calls and telegrams Keffer was persuaded to authorize the release of a quantity of the drug from Squibb Labs in New Brunswick, New Jersey. A police escort raced with the dying child's doctor to the lab where they obtained the drug and rushed back to the city. After two days on an intravenous penicillin drip the child was dramatically improved. In six weeks she was back home.[1]

Mass production was one of the main obstacles to the widespread use of penicillin. This problem was solved in time for the D-Day invasion thanks to a process of deep tank fermentation devised by a small Brooklyn, NY company, Charles Pfizer & Co., and a chemical engineer named Jasper Kane. In March 1943, Kane began experimenting with 14 7,500-gallon tanks and by the end of the year the company had mass-produced over 45 million units of penicillin. On June 6, 1944, 90% of allied soldiers were carrying a dose of the antibiotic produced in Brooklyn.[2] [3]

The second significant obstacle to the mass application of penicillin was the short-term effect of a single dose. In 1945, penicillin pioneer Alexander Fleming (1881-1955) was touring the US Walter Reed Army Medical Center where virtually every soldier had been injected with penicillin. While there, Fleming learned of two army doctors who had solved the dose duration problem by administering penicillin in a mixture of peanut oil and beeswax.

US Army Medical Corps Captain Monroe J. Romansky (1911-2006) had discovered a method of prolonging the action of penicillin by mixing it with 4% to 4.8% beeswax and peanut oil to create POB (penicillin in oil-beeswax) also known as the Romansky Formula.[4] The mix was a viscous, butter-like substance that was difficult to draw up into the syringe.[5]

It was a simple solution to the problem. The peanut oil in the POB coated the penicillin particles. As the body metabolized the oil, the drug was released slowly into the system. The formula extended the dose from three hours to single daily injections. The Romansky Formula became a standard in the manufacture of penicillin from that moment on. For this discovery, President Truman awarded the doctor the Legion of Merit.

Penicillin POB actually doubled penicillin blood levels according to research at the Montreal General Hospital in 1947. But this success was not without side effects. The amount of beeswax and oil used was reduced "in an attempt to eliminate undesirable reactions".[6] And in 1950, a study of penicillin treatments in over 100 children at the Philadelphia Children's Hospital reported additional obstacles to the formula. The Romansky Formula had created peanut allergy in an undisclosed number of children:

> Although good clinical results were reported, certain
> disadvantages were encountered, namely, difficulty in
> administration, variability of absorption, local pain at the
> site of injection, sensitivity to peanut oil or beeswax, and
> sterile abscess formation.[7]

Iatrogenic side effects including allergy from penicillin injections were "distinct hazards".[8] Because of this, doctors at the World Health Organisation were alarmed at the overuse and misuse of the drug. In 1953, 600 tons of penicillin, streptomycin and broad-spectrum antibiotics were produced.[9] [10] Their widespread application had resulted in fatal anaphylaxis, antibiotic resistant bacterial strains, fungal overgrowth and gastro-intestinal dysbiosis.[11]

An estimated 2.5% of all children injected with penicillin developed an allergy to it.

In 1948, doctors also began to use PAM (penicillin with aluminium monostearate) an aqueous solution again suspended in peanut oil. PAM was much easier to administer than POB and it produced desirable penicillin blood-levels for 24 to 26 hours. PAM was recommended by the WHO for control of syphilis, yaws (a tropical infection of bones and joints caused by spirochete bacterium) and other infections. By the end of 1957, approximately 35 million people had been injected with the peanut oil based PAM.[12]

Allergic reactivity dogged PAM as well. For at least one doctor, the mass allergic reaction to penicillin reminded him of "serum sickness of former days".[13] In 1953, the media warned of increased "peril" from penicillin. Severe and fatal reactions were being reported with increasing frequency.[14]

In essence, the use of penicillin had created a mass allergic phenomenon with anaphylactic fatalities.[15] And since the US had the highest rate of consumption of penicillin in the world at this time, the majority of fatalities to the drug were reported there. Between 1% and 10% of the US population was allergic to penicillin in 2009 – the wide range attributed to insufficient formal study yielding to anecdotal reports.

It was important that the peanut oil used in penicillin was refined to remove as much of the sensitizing peanut proteins as possible. However, not only was it impossible to remove all the proteins[16] but also the quality of refinement varied between makers.[17] On this basis in 2000, an expert committee on labeling at the WHO resisted giving a full endorsement to the oil.[18] Investigations had shown that refined peanut oil in foods had both sensitized and caused allergic reactions in children.[19] [20] Refined peanut oil can create allergy whether consumed or injected.

While some people injected with POB became peanut allergic, it was a seemingly infrequent development at this time. And because it appeared to be relatively safe in single injections, peanut oil acquired a history of acceptable use. It became a reasonable choice for inclusion in many other injectable drugs.[21] [22] [23] It was subsequently used as a base for injected epinephrine for children with asthma[24] and as an adjuvant in vaccines for tetanus.[25] It was used in oral drugs.[26] Unknown to the consumer, peanut oil became a popular ingredient in injected and oral medications, vitamins, skin creams, infant formula and more.[27]

Why peanut?
Peanut oil was a natural choice for Romansky. Peanuts were homegrown, tariff protected, relatively inexpensive, plentiful, remained stable in heat for long periods without going rancid[28] and above all, they were not rationed during the

war. During war and in times of scarcity – the Civil War, both World Wars and the Great Depression – Americans had turned to peanut and peanut oil as substitutes for food, medicine and fuel.

Romansky had few oils from which to choose in creating his formula. All imports of oil (especially coconut oil which was most stable in heat) from the Philippines and British colonies in Asia were cut off after the bombing of Pearl Harbor. And cottonseed oil, the only other contender for home grown excipient that had been a favorite before the war, was unreliable. There was suspicion that refined cottonseed oil being produced at the time was not free of sensitizing proteins and that it was toxic.

The cottonseed industry had been weakened by bad deals and bad luck. As previously discussed, the 1909-1920 boll weevil blight that precipitated an agricultural crisis in 1919, was only the beginning of misfortune for cottonseed. The Crash of 1929 was followed by a drought from 1929-39 that forced cotton farmers from the land. When they did return, it was to grow peanuts. Peanuts were suited to the same soil as cotton and appeared more resistant to insects.

During the US Civil War when the northern blockade prevented the import of goods by the south, peanut and peanut oil were used as substitutes for innumerable essentials. Peanut oil was a superior replacement for whale oil to lubricate machinery because it didn't smoke.[29] It was used extensively as a lubricant for railroad locomotives, wood and cotton spindles. Cooks substituted peanut oil for lard – lard, especially from pork, was the preferred frying medium in the US. In fact, pigs were fed peanut and allowed to run in the fields to route them up.[30] Confederacy army cooks used peanuts extensively in cooking as malnutrition and hunger persisted through the war. Peanuts substituted for coffee and were used as recipe fillers. Recipes were created for peanut drinks, peanut pie, peanut sausage and peanut mayonnaise.

But as the Civil War ended so too did the large scale emergency manufacture of peanut oil. Attempts to re-ignite the peanut industry post-war were not wholly successful and the limited demand for the oil was satisfied by German imports made from peanuts grown in their African colonies. With the outbreak of another war, WWI, this import from Germany ceased.

At the same time, however, the demand for peanut oil skyrocketed. Peanut, the wartime substitute was needed even more desperately in the form of glycerin when the US entered WW I in 1917. Glycerin was used to make explosives. To meet the sudden demand, peanut oil mills sprang up through the south and cultivation of the legume increased to 4,000,000 acres on land formerly used for cotton.

In the US, peanuts became closely aligned with war. They were so much a part of wartime that eating and growing them became patriotic acts. "Peanuts and Patriotism" a 1917 article in *The Forum* exclaimed that peanuts served valiantly in the war effort by conserving dairy products, substituting for meat and feeding livestock.[31] And the National Emergency Food Garden Commission encouraged even small gardeners to grow them.

During the Great War, peanuts became one of the most important commercial crops in the US. But with the close of the war, cheap peanut imports flooded the US and domestic prices plummeted. Needing government intervention to regain control of the market, a suffering peanut industry turned to the influential agricultural chemist George Washington Carver (1864-1943).

Carver knew of 30,117 uses for peanut.[32] He had developed a host of products with peanut including axle grease, adhesives, cosmetics, linoleum, metal polish, shaving cream, wood stain and a vitalizing skin rub for polio victims.[33] Carver patented several of his peanut discoveries including a formula for Penol. Penol was cough syrup made from an emulsion of peanut juices and creosote.

In 1921, Carver was asked to speak as an expert witness before the House Ways and Means Committee on behalf of the United Peanut Growers' Association. The group was seeking tariff protection from the flood of peanuts and peanut oil coming from China and Japan. At the hearing Carver began by presenting his "Pandora's Box" filled with 101 peanut products.[34] Initially allotted only 10 minutes, Carver spoke for an hour and forty minutes as he presented peanut candies, cakes, peanut "milk", mock meats, breakfast foods, shoe polish and wood stains. The committee applauded his valuable contributions to science. At his second presentation to the Finance Committee Carver's plea on behalf of the peanut industry was successful. With a tariff in place, peanut imports began to decline.

This tariff protection set the peanut industry up for a boom and World War II created the opportunity for it to happen. During this war, the per capital consumption of peanuts and peanut products almost doubled due to shortages of other foods, the non-rationing of peanuts and lack of competition from imported and domestic nuts and oils. In 1942, *Fortune Magazine* claimed that 600 million pounds of peanut oil would need to be produced for food and, again in wartime, for glycerin in the manufacture of explosives.[35] The Secretary of Agriculture launched the "Food for Freedom" program in 1943, telling farmers they needed to plant 5.5 million acres of peanuts. The peanut could win the war and sustain them in peacetime.[36]

Through WW II, the peanut industry doubled in size and prices were two to three times higher than before the war. By 1944 twice as much land was utilized than before the war to produce 2.5 billion pounds of peanuts worth $200,000,000.[37] The equivalent in 2009 would be about $24.5 Billion.

Determined that this boom in peanut sales would not end, the US National Peanut Council threw money at increasing public consumption of the legume. The Council proposed to spend $1,000,000 over three years to find new uses for the peanut, to study insect infestation control, and to promote the peanut's role in American life. Industry leaders were also concerned that the government market protections might be eliminated. Although the industry had never been stronger and it was reported that Americans ate more peanuts than any other people, the council president Walter Richards stated, "our present situation is dangerous and may lead to a serious crisis."[38]

By Jan. 1945, a *New York Times* reporter wrote that a shortage of peanuts loomed. And in Oct. 1945, the retail prices of peanut butter increased by six cents per pound. The Peanut and Nut Salters Association warned of a shortage of civilian supplies of peanut predicting a 50% cut.[39] But the fears were unfounded. By 1947, there was a "whopper" crop and exports had climbed to 45% of the total peanut market.[40] Government subsidized grants and loans had helped cushion the transition from wartime to peacetime.[41] In 1950, 2,200,000 acres were allotted to this crop producing two billion pounds of peanuts.[42]

Peanut oil in the manufacture of penicillin POB was an easy choice for Romansky during WW II. It was available during wartime, stable in heat, relatively inexpensive and patriotic. While the exact number of people made peanut allergic are unknown for the post-war years, they were likely low and cut across all demographics. Injected penicillin was administered to adults and children alike.

Articles published in 1956, 1961 and 1963[43] reflected a growing awareness of the allergy in medical circles but there was no impact from this on pubic consumption or on peanut industry revenues.

In fact, the peanut industry continued to experience growth. In the 1970s, the unprecedented demand following the election of peanut farmer President Jimmy Carter (1977-81) was like winning the lottery. The themed presidency of "Peanut One" spurred soaring consumption of peanuts and peanut butter in schools and a bonanza for growers.[44] Testament to power of the peanut industry was the continued support of government when the 1995 Farm Bill challenged farmer subsidies. Peanut friendly government representatives ensured that supply management was again secured in law for the all American crop.[45]

The peanut industry remained strong until a marked decline in the 1990s when the peanut allergy epidemic took a bite out of its bottom line. Between 1993 and 1999, the peanut's share of the snack foods market fell from 14.4% to 12.4%.[46] Of a $21.6 Billion industry in 2006, this drop represented a significant loss[47] of about $432 Million in annual gross revenues. The important consumer category of children under 14 was in decline.

Peanut oil in vaccines

In 1964, the *New York Times*[48] announced that pharmaceutical giant Merck had begun to use a new vaccine ingredient that promised to extend immunity against influenza, polio and other illnesses.[49] This new ingredient patented just four days earlier was called Adjuvant 65-4.[50] It contained up to 65% peanut oil as well as Arlacel A, aluminum stearate and other ingredients. The *Times* article explained the impressive value of the peanut oil in the adjuvant that was similar to its action in penicillin. The oil surrounds the vaccine antigens. When the vaccine is injected into the muscle, the oil is gradually metabolised by the body providing a sustained release of the other ingredients.[51]

Adjuvant 65 had been a six-year research effort between Merck and the Children's Hospital of Philadelphia, the same hospital in which experiments using the Romansky Formula on children had resulted in peanut allergies. In 1966, Merck introduced this novel peanut oil additive to the public in a flu vaccine.[52]

An adjuvant (from the Latin "adjuvare" to enhance) is a vaccine additive that stimulates the body's production of antibodies to a viral or bacterial antigen. In the 1930s, American immunologist Jules Freund (1890-1960) created an adjuvant by mixing aluminum mineral salts with mycobacteria in emulsified mineral oil.[53] Freund's complete adjuvant (FCA) was quickly withdrawn, however, and banned from use in humans because of its toxic side effects. FCA produced granulomas, abscesses, and autoimmune diseases. According to writer Gary Matsumoto, Freund himself had warned that animals injected with his adjuvant developed severe allergic conditions such as allergic aspermatogenesis (loss of sperm production), experimental allergic encephalomyelitis (MS) and allergic neuritis (leading to paralysis). The oil in water emulsion without added mycobacteria is known as Freund's incomplete adjuvant (FIA) and, being less toxic, was used in human vaccines. Mineral oil adjuvants are no longer used in humans in the US and many other countries.

Thus the arrival of Adjuvant 65 meant hope for the creation of safer and more widely distributed vaccines. Previous experiments with other adjuvants in flu vaccines had had limited success. In a 1964 British study of over 900 subjects (allergic subjects were excluded) shot with a flu vaccine, one subject was incapacitated and several others actually developed the flu resulting in consumer resistance to the products.[54] These vaccine designs did not, as was hoped, incite a "desire for re-vaccination".

Next to such failures, the introduction of Adjuvant 65-4 in a flu vaccine in the late 1960s was seen as an improvement.[55] Several medical journal articles

PEANUT OIL USED IN A NEW VACCINE

Product Patented for Merck Said to Extend Immunity

By STACY V. JONES
Special to The New York Times

WASHINGTON, Sept. 18 —A pharmaceutical manufacturer has developed a vaccine that it predicts will considerably lengthen immunity from influenza and other virus infections, thereby requiring fewer "shots."

The key ingredient, called Adjuvant 65, which contains peanut oil, was patented this week for Merck & Co., Inc., by Dr. Allen F. Woodhour and Dr. Thomas B. Stim. They discovered it in the company's research laboratory at West Point, Pa.

Present procedure, according to Merck, is to give annual injections of killed influenza virus, which are expected to afford protection for a year. The hope is that the new vaccine will extend the immunity to at least two years and be more effective during that period.

The current issue of the New England Journal of Medicine reports favorably on studies in which 880 persons received killed influenza virus in Adjuvant 65.

Still Under Study

The new vaccine is still under study and is not yet licensed for general use.

Adjuvant slowly releases antigens, the active ingredients of vaccines, which stimulate the creation of antibodies in the human system over an extended period, Merck said.

Adjuvant is an emulsion of refined peanut oil in water to which are added an emulsifier and a stabilizer.

As the company explains it, the antigens are contained in small particles of water, which are surrounded by the oil. When injected into the body, the emulsion is distributed along the muscle fibers. The antigens are released as the peanut oil is absorbed by the body's tissues.

The research on Adjuvant covered six years and represented the collaboration of several departments of the Merck Institute for Therapeutic Research and the Children's Hospital of Philadelphia.

Dr. Woodhour is assistant director of the department of virus diseases in the Merck laboratories. Dr. Stim is now a research associate at Yale University. Their patent is No. 3,149,036.

Stacy V. Jones, "Peanut oil used in new vaccine; product patented for Merck said to extend immunity," *The New York Times*, Business Financial Section (Sept. 19, 1964) 31.

123

published in the early 1970s extolled the effectiveness of this peanut oil adjuvant that produced extremely high antibody levels. The adjuvant showed a level of antibodies that was 13 fold higher than that produced by an aqueous medium.[56]

Adjuvant 65 had the potential to become an important addition to any vaccine. One of its inventors who had patented Adjuvant 65 with Merck, Maurice Hilleman (1919-2005)[57] helped write a report as a member of the WHO Scientific Group on Immunological Adjuvants. The report published in 1973, explained that this peanut oil additive had resulted in: elevated antibody titres; elevated titres for sustained periods; a broad antigenic response; and reduced cost of production because adjuvants were antigen sparing. With an adjuvant, vaccines needed less of the expensive antigen to achieve a superior stimulation of the immune system. In addition, vegetable oil was easier to metabolize than mineral oil.[58] The mineral oil adjuvant "potentiates allergic responses".[59]

But so too could Adjuvant 65.

Hilleman and the expert group knew of the danger of injected proteins. The group conceded that any breakage of the peanut emulsions in the body, "especially when allergens are employed" was dangerous. As well it was important with oil adjuvants that the injection be administered deep into the muscle "since there is a far greater chance of adverse effects when they are deposited subcutaneously". Doctors and nurses must be carefully trained, they warned, in the art of deep muscular injection and that "they should appreciate the need for it in this context."[60]

Injection into the bloodstream would virtually guarantee allergic sensitization to peanut or any other extant vaccine proteins.

Noting that Adjuvant 65 was prepared using "highly refined arachis oil" and that within two months it was almost completely metabolised, the chance of any harmful effects was reduced. The report confirmed that, "No sensitization to the components of the adjuvant, including peanut oil, occurred."

Hilleman and his colleagues knew that allergic sensitization to the peanut oil in this adjuvant was a distinct possibility.

Again, it was impossible to remove all protein from peanut oil. According to the FDA, the amount of peanut protein in the refined oil varied by manufacturer, processes used and by tests used to detect it. Trace levels of intact proteins would always remain.[61]

The Romansky Formula had created peanut allergy. And as it turned out, oil in water adjuvants like Adjuvant 65 too could create allergy to "contaminant proteins" in flu vaccines.

In 1973, an article on the role of adjuvant using peanut oil in flu vaccines was specifically observed to create "untoward" hypersensitivity to the proteins in the vaccine.[62] Adjuvants were hard to control in the body and caused delayed hypersensitivity reactions. "Trouble" lay with the oils and emulsifiers being "insufficiently characterized", stated one researcher:

> An adjuvant will indiscriminately augment immune
> reactions, particularly delayed hypersensitivity reactions,
> against all the contaminant proteins and lipoproteins as
> well as against the virus antigens.[63]

Tension existed between reports prepared by Hilleman at the WHO and those in the medical literature regarding the relative safety of adjuvants. Mounting concerns in the medical literature regarding allergy echoed those expressed in the media following one of the first profiled peanut allergy deaths in the US. In 1972, a child in Boston died after eating peanut butter ice cream.

Doctors acknowledged the rising prevalence of peanut allergy. In 1973, S.A. Bock began the first US study of 114 peanut allergic children.

By 1974, the peanut oil based Adjuvant 65 was licensed for general use in the UK[64] but had failed to obtain approval in the US. And so, Hilleman helped develop several other patented formulations of the same basic adjuvant attempting to satisfy government requirements.[65] It appeared that what made it effective, certain "undefined impurities", were blocking its approval. In the US, the only stand-alone adjuvant approved by the FDA was aluminum salt (alum). The policy of the FDA was to approve adjuvants as they appeared within a complete vaccine formula. Vaccine formulae were approved with peanut oil adjuvants but not with Adjuvant 65 as a stand-alone product.

Ultimately, the company decided not to pursue Adjuvant 65 any further in the US.[66] According to one author, a subsequent review of the safety of Adjuvant 65 over 10 years published in 1973, showed that Arlacel A in the emulsified peanut oil adjuvant appeared to induce tumors in mice. Some believed that it was this adverse effect that had kept the formula from receiving license.[67]

Extreme caution followed the introduction of the water-in-oil adjuvants. The mechanism for alum's tendency to stimulate eosinophilia and enhance IgE production was unknown, but its consequence was an undeniable increase in allergenicity and neurotoxicity.[68] [69] [70] [71] A seminal review of adjuvanted vaccines in 1980 cautioned that these vaccine additives should not risk induction of allergy or other iatrogenic illnesses.[72]

The challenge in vaccine adjuvant design was to gain potency while minimizing toxicity.[73]   And many doctors saw toxicity and allergenicity as acceptable compromises in vaccination goals.   In a student textbook published in 2000, one author was critical of a colleague who believed that "any toxicity that we accept is a compromise."   This compromise, stated the author, "must become an accepted principle in the search for adjuvants suitable for use in human vaccines because one of their functions is to stimulate antigen presenting cells."[74]

In the late 1970s and 1980s, Adjuvant 65 was not eligible for use in US vaccines. However, it did become a model for other adjuvants.   Based on Hilleman's precedent setting formula, one researcher published on a Novel Lipid Emulsion adjuvant using peanut oil for use in humans.[75]   As well, Adjuvant 65 was a precedent cited in many vaccine patents using emulsified peanut oil adjuvants. The general use of peanut in vaccines became common practice.[76] [77] [78]

Adjuvants, revealed immunologist Charles Janeway (1943-2003) a Howard Hughes Medical Institute investigator and Yale University School of Medicine professor in 1989, were the "immunologists' dirty little secret".   The secret was really a poorly understood puzzle regarding the body's response to them.[79] Janeway suggested that there are cross-reactive combinations of which researchers are unaware but which the body recognises.[80]

The difficult balance between potency and safety had long been recognized in vaccine design.   In fact, a competitive edge between vaccine makers had been found on either side of the issues of efficacy and side effects.

CEO of BioVant Stephen Simes was quoted in a 2006 business article.   In the article, the CEO was quoted as distinguishing his company's products from those of its competitors in the vaccine market based on their lower rate of allergy inducing side effects.   He was quoted to have said that the problem with most adjuvants was that they could cause allergies and those of BioVant brand, while not as potent as others were safer.[81]

Vaccines can create allergies. And peanut, as discussed in Chapter 3, is more allergenic than other substances. It has been suggested that the peanut has adjuvant properties of its own that make it "a perfect allergen".[82] The "hydrophobic" residues of the amino acids in Ara h 1 peanut epitope are protected within the structure of the protein from degradation by digestion.[83] Indeed, an "allergenic" feature of proteins is their stability when heated or processed.

Given the resilience of peanut proteins, peanut oil appeared to have been a poor choice for inclusion in an aluminum-based adjuvant intended to excite an immune response.

The slow rise of peanut allergy began after the introduction of Romansky's peanut oil and beeswax formula in penicillin. A growing prevalence came with the use of peanut oil in a range of pharmaceuticals including the Adjuvant 65-4 inspired progeny after 1964. Peanut allergy studies were launched in the 1970s followed by sporadic deaths from peanut allergy and increasing media attention.

And so doctors watched the slowly rising prevalence of peanut allergy, none publicly posing the obvious questions – like the cottonseed oil mystery of the 1930s and 40s, how were people being sensitized to this food in the first place?

Of significance in this new allergy mystery, however, was its specific impact on children. It may have seemed coincidental that the disproportionate numbers of adjuvanted vaccines containing peanut oil were administered to children during routine vaccination.

Peanut allergy acceleration

In the early 1990s, a sudden surge of peanut allergic four and five year old children filled school systems across Canada, the UK and the US. It caught many educators off guard.[84] Eyewitness accounts of this phenomenon confirmed by ER admission records and two UK studies of preschoolers point to this moment – prevalence of peanut allergy in children suddenly accelerated around 1990.

Functionally, there are a limited number of ways in which a person can become anaphylactic to any substance – ingestion, inhalation, through the skin and injection. And historically, the only mechanism implicated in mass allergy – from serum sickness to penicillin – was injection. Further, this period of allergy acceleration correlated to an unprecedented series of political, social, legal and economic reforms directed at childhood vaccinations. Swift, identical alterations to the pediatric vaccination schedules of Canada, the UK, the US, Australia and many other western countries occurred simultaneously between the late 1980s and early 1990s.

The peanut allergy epidemic was precipitated by vaccination. Events leading up to it unfolded in plain sight.

In the spring of 1985, 231 lawsuits were pending in the US against four vaccine manufacturers.[85] Vaccine makers were paying out millions of dollars in settlements, their legal defense costs soared and insurance was becoming prohibitive. Previously, courts had declared that vaccine makers could not be held strictly liable for selling products "with a known but apparently reasonable risk."[86] The doctors and parents were deemed largely responsible for the risk and any ensuing damage. But as injuries mounted suits against manufacturers were allowed based on a "failure to warn". During the flu non-epidemic of 1976, emergency vaccines administered to about 45 million people over three months were linked to a significant rise in Guillain-Barré Syndrome.[87] These and other side effects resulted in more than 4,000 complaints settled by the US government for $72 million.[88]

This event opened the door to a flood of vaccine related lawsuits – cases involving the DPT vaccine escalated from one suit in 1979 to 255 in 1986. Vaccine maker Lederle estimated that total sales of its 1983 polio vaccine were only one-twelfth the value of claims filed against it.[89]

In this litigious environment, many pharmaceutical companies simply abandoned the vaccine market leaving the US supply in the hands of a few makers. Even the pharmaceutical giant Merck was challenged in 1979 by an internal report questioning their continued presence in vaccine research and development.[90] By 1985, the US was facing a vaccine shortage that threatened public health, declared a report published by US Institute of Medicine (IOM).[91]

To reduce the uncertainty faced by manufacturers, the IOM called for the federal government to provide "equitable, rapid compensation in a consistent fashion". In 1986, President Reagan signed the National Childhood Vaccine Injury Act from which emerged the Vaccine Injury Compensation Program (VICP) in 1988. VICP was a "no fault" alternative to the tort system in which eligible claims would be determined by a federal court and paid by the federal government.[92] Until parents had first exhausted this approach, their tort claims could not proceed. In this new legal environment, the pressures on vaccine makers eased.[93] The number of pending lawsuits quickly dropped to just a handful.

But US public health was perceived to be in danger from yet another source: parents who were slow to vaccinate their children before the start of school.

The vaccination rate for pre-school children under four years of age in 1985 was between 55% and 65%.[94]   Obstacles to vaccination were cost for many but inconvenience for more: there were seven vaccines in 1985. The schedule included two combination vaccines, measles-mumps-rubella (MMR) and diphtheria pertussis-tetanus (DPT) plus a multi-strain oral polio vaccine (OPV). Parents typically put off vaccination until their children reached school age, by which time and with school requirements, 90% of all children were fully vaccinated.

Therefore in 1991, the Bush government took action on a goal of raising national vaccination levels among preschool children to 90% by the year 2000. Vaccination action plans were formulated by all states and 28 metropolitan areas. Federal grant funds were authorized for direct delivery of vaccination services as well as vaccine purchase. New awards for state grants tripled from $37 Million in 1991 to $98.2 Million in 1993.

The US strategy focused on preschool children was on course with the World Health Organization's 1974 Expanded Programme on Immunization. The WHO's global strategy was to achieve 80-90% Universal Childhood Immunization with a wide range of vaccines through all national systems in all countries throughout the world.[95] Other international vaccination endeavors included the Children's Vaccine Initiative launched in New York City in 1990. This program added to the vaccination pressure aimed at all children in the hardest to reach and poorest places of the world.[96]

In 1985, the US government had established disease priorities. The IOM had proposed a ranking system to determine the ongoing "diseases of importance"[97] based on: the expected health benefits to be achieved by reducing morbidity and mortality to the specific disease; and the anticipated net savings of health care resources. This model was applied to 14 diseases in the US resulting in a top five: Hep B; respiratory syncytial virus (RSV); Haemophilus influenzae type b (Hib); influenza; herpesvirus varicellae (for "high risk" individuals). This government study concluded that the creation of a Hib vaccine was a high priority need – giving direction for innovation to pharmaceutical companies.

When this decision was made the novel conjugate Hib specifically formulated for infants was already in development.[98] [99]

Hib is a bacterium that can cause meningitis, an inflammation of the membranes covering the spinal cord and brain. While it had been successfully treated in the past with antibiotics, the bacterium was becoming resistant to this treatment. According to research, the pathogen was responsible for the majority of systemic infections in children in 1981.[100] An estimated .5% of all US children developed a Hib infection[101] and 5%[102] of these (.025% of all children) would die from complications of the disease. However, US national mortality rates for Hib were already naturally decreasing between 1980 and 1987, an average of 8.5% each year. Between 1988 and 1991, mortality to the disease decreased by 48%.[103] This rapid drop was credited to the introduction of Hib vaccines.

The PRP (Haemophilus b polysacchardide, polyribosylribitol phosphate) vaccine for Hib was licensed in April 1985 in the US for children over two years of age. While it was not without concerns during clinical trials,[104] PRP was used by Praxis in the manufacture of b Capsa 1, by Lederle in HibImmune and by Connaught in HibVAX.

However, responsiveness to PRP was age dependent. It was ineffective in children under 18 months of age and had variable effects in two year olds.[105] A solution to this was already in development – the conjugate vaccine.

The bacteria for which conjugated vaccines are designed have an important structural feature in common. They are surrounded by a thick and slippery capsule. The Hib capsule is made of carbohydrate and provides a target for attack by the immune system. Antibodies to the carbohydrate can bind to the capsule and enable the white blood cells to destroy the bacterium.

However, the immune systems of children under two years of age do not respond to carbohydrate antigens. Because of this fact, a vaccine was created that linked the carbohydrate antigen with a toxic carrier protein to which an infant's system could respond.[106] The conjugate vaccine for Hib consisted of a toxic carrier protein (tetanus or diphtheria toxoids) that was covalently bound to some aspect of the bacterium (ie. its membrane proteins): a chemical process bonded these two molecules covalently.

The first protein-conjugated Hib vaccine using a protein carrier diphtheria toxoid (polyribosylribitol-diphtheria toxoid PRP-D) was branded as ProHibit by Connaught. It was licensed on Dec. 22, 1987 for children 18 months and older. It was re-licensed in Dec. 1989 for 15-month-old children.

The FDA licensed this vaccine based on a Finnish trial in which 30,000 children were injected with the PRP-D. It showed 83% effectiveness but 20 children suffered serious adverse reactions. Another study challenged the efficacy of the PRP-D stating it actually made babies more susceptible to invasive Hib in the window shortly after injection and up to three weeks following administration.[107] The vaccine appeared to depress the immune system.

Other licensed variations of the same conjugate concept quickly flooded the market. As they did, the age limit for their administration quickly dropped for most brands from two years to two months of age:

- Dec. 20, 1989, conjugated Hib vaccine PedvaxHIB by Merck was licensed using PRP-OMP OMP (PRP conjugated with outer membrane protein of Neisseria meningitides) for routine vaccination at 15 months of age. On Dec. 13, 1990, this brand was re-licensed for two-month-old children.

- Oct. 4, 1990, the first of a series of Hib vaccines for two month old children appeared, Hib-TITER by Lederie-Praxis. The vaccine used HbOC, a Hib oligosaccharide bonded to a diphtheria toxoid.

- PRP-CRM another conjugate formulation using protein CRM197, a mutant diphtheriae protein. It had been previously licensed for 18 month olds (Dec. 22, 1988); 15 month olds (Dec. 1989) and finally licensed for two month old children in 1990.

- March 30, 1993, PRP-T by Pasteur Merieux-Connaught Vaccins in ActHIB used a tetanus toxoid as protein carrier licensed for use on two-month-old children.[108]

In four years, five Hib vaccines were licensed to different companies. These vaccines were marketed, sold to governments and administered to consumers under the age of two.

These vaccines differed in the molecular size of the Hib polysaccharide, the toxic protein used as the carrier, and the methods used to link the polysaccharide to the protein. Thus, according to the IOM in 1994, it is "plausible that variations in the type or frequency of adverse effects may occur because of the differences in the polysaccharide or protein components of the vaccines."[109]

An additional challenge existed in that the Hib vaccine was to be administered at the same time as DPT and polio (OPV). ActHIB, by design, had to be reconstituted by and therefore administered with, the combination diphtheria and tetanus toxoids and acellular pertussis vaccine.[110] The vaccines were combined for convenience.   One shot saved time for parents and reduced the child's discomfort.[111]   Doctors blended these vaccines together drawing them literally into the same syringe from different vials and then injecting this mixture into the infant.

Before the FDA licensed this blend, however, a study was conducted on a group of approximately 5,000 Navajo children between July 1988 and Aug. 1990.   One report showed efficacy of 90% for PRP-outer membrane protein vaccine (PRP-OMP) in Navajo infants when given at two and four months of age and 100 percent after three doses of oligosaccharide conjugate Hib (HbOC) vaccine given at two, four, and six months of age.[112]

Another non-government report described the results very differently.   Half of the Navajo babies were vaccinated with five vaccines at once, Hib PRP-OMP, DPT and OPV, and the other half given a placebo with DPT and OPV.   Two doses were given with follow up time of about 270 days.   What followed was an outbreak of Hib influenza within the both groups in 1990.   23 cases were reported.   Surprisingly, 22 of these infections were in the placebo group.   Other infections were reported in both groups and 16 deaths, according to the non-government report.[113]

By 1991, more than 17 million doses of Hib were sold in the US alone.   It was a revenue generating "blockbuster product" according to a 1998 WHO publication.[114]   Whether or not there was a general consensus in the medical community regarding the need for extensive use of this vaccine,[115] it seemed that its application had led to a general decline in prevalence of the influenza infection in children under five.[116]   The human cost of building this immunity, however, was not widely discussed.

With speed and efficiency, the US pediatric vaccination strategy intensified. In 1992, additional doses of combination vaccines were included in the schedule.[117] Between 1993 and 1995 the Clinton administration's Childhood Immunization Initiative provided federal funds for service, delivery and immunization programs that peaked at $261 million in state and local awards in 1995. The government's 1994 "National Vaccine Plan"[118] aimed at 90% coverage of all infants. To that end, the Vaccines for Children Program was adopted as an amendment to Medicaid (1994) providing about $500 million in federal funds for vaccine purchase and delivery. Vaccination also became a requirement before entry to many preschools and day cares.

By 1997-98, childhood vaccination coverage rates reached record highs.[119] The pharmaceutical industry had estimated gross sales of US$100 Billion in the mid-1980s.[120] By 2008, it was an estimated US$500 Billion with the market shared by a small number of companies.

Other westernized countries adopted a schedule similar to that of the US as recommended by the World Health Organization (6, 10 and 14 weeks). In Australia, PRP-D, ProHIBIT was licensed in 1992 for infants 18 months of age. By 1993, HBOC (HibTITER), PRP-T (Act-HIB) and PRP-OMP (PedvaxHIB) were licensed for routine vaccination of infants starting at two months.[121]

In Canada, starting in 1987, a similar progression was made through the Hib vaccines – HbOC (HibTiter), PRP-OMP (PedVaxHIB), PRP-T (tetanus toxoid, ActHIB) and PRP-D (diphtheria toxoid, ProHIBit) in conjunction with MMR, DPT and polio at this time. The compulsory Canadian Immunization of School Pupils Act was amended to include exemptions in 1984 following protests from the Committee Against Compulsory Vaccination. From then on, parents could obtain vaccination exemptions for medical or ethical reasons, but few did so.

Vaccination rates according to WHO data were between 90% and 96% in 1993 and remained high.

The UK also adopted the WHO policies introducing Hib conjugate in the pediatric schedule in 1992.[122] Like the Canadian statistics, the UK rates in 1990 were 89% to 90% vaccination coverage and remained above 90% through the 1990s.

In 1993, DPT and Hib were included in the first licensed four-vaccines-in-one-needle. The first was Tetramune by Lederle. This was followed by OmniHIB from Pasteur Merieux Vaccins.

In 1994, five vaccines were packaged into a single needle. The first was PENTA (DPT-Polio-Hib PRP-T) by Connaught (North American arm of Institut Merieux of France later bought by Aventis).[123]

According to the CDC, combination vaccines reduced the number of injections, improved vaccination timeliness and coverage and reduced shipping and storage costs. Disadvantages were the potential for increased adverse events, extra doses of antigen needed to achieve required antibody levels and reduced effectiveness for certain ages.[124] Doctors admitted that unforeseeable incompatibilities when different antigens and chemicals were combined into one vaccine were distinct concerns.[125] [126] [127]

Starting at two months of age infants were being administered vaccines that had been hastily produced and mixed with other vaccines without the benefit of longitudinal studies.[128] The unprecedented schedule had been shaped by political and economic imperatives and made smooth by legal reforms that relieved pharmaceutical companies of any serious liability if something went wrong. It was a perfect storm of international programs and goals that would have negative implications for certain children and their unwary parents.

During this period of expanding pediatric vaccination in western countries, the prevalence of peanut and other food allergies in children accelerated. Unseen by the public, hospital ER records in Australia, the UK and the US documented the upward momentum of food anaphylaxis admissions for children under five. In the US, ER records showed a steady and rapid increase in anaphylaxis discharges between 1992 and 1994 from 467 per 100,000 to 671. This number jumped to 876 in 1995.[129] In three years between 1992 and 1995 the numbers had nearly doubled. A 1991 US study determined that 90% of all food allergy fatalities were due to ingestion of peanut/tree nuts.[130] The Isle of Wight studies revealed a dramatic doubling of peanut allergy in preschool children in just four years rising from .5% in 1994 to 1.1% in 1998.

The same phenomenon occurred in the US. In 1997 .6% of American children were allergic to peanut. By 2002, this number had doubled to 1.2%.

In those five years, the peanut allergic pediatric population in the US alone grew by an average of 90,960 children a year.[131]

Part 3

PEANUT ALLERGY AT THE CROSSOVER POINT

Chapter 6

Absorbing the Costs

Ingredients

Vaccination was the elephant in the room. Researchers glanced at it, knew it was there but were reluctant to get too close. Only a handful of doctors at the time looked directly at vaccination and asked whether a reduction of common childhood diseases through a policy of mass vaccination was worth the price of a higher prevalence of allergy and other adverse outcomes.[1]

Vaccines are a complex blend of antigens, stabilizers, adjuvants, preservatives, anti-bacterials, anti-fungals, suspending fluids, gels and more. While manufacturers, government and doctors are not obliged to reveal the precise ingredients of vaccines, the CDC offered a limited list.[2] The common childhood vaccine DtaP-IPV/Hib (Pentacel), for example, contains: aluminum phosphate, bovine serum albumin, formaldehyde, glutaraldhyde, MRC-5 DNA and cellular protein, neomycin, polymyxin b sulfate, polysorbate 80, 2-phenoxyethanol. MRC-5 (Medical Research Council 5) is a cell line developed in 1966 from lung tissue taken from a 14-week-old fetus aborted for psychiatric reason from a 27-year-old woman, and more. Bovine serum albumin (BSA) is blood protein from cattle. Neomycin is an antibiotic. Aluminum phosphate is part of an antigen sparing adjuvant.

Adjuvants, as already discussed, stimulate the immune system to respond to just a small amount of antigen. They reduce the cost of a vaccine and increase its efficacy measured in antibodies specific to the disease being addressed. However, they can be dangerous. The choice of adjuvant (or even whether to use one or not) in any vaccine by a maker or government reflects a compromise between immune stimulation and invariable side effects that would be produced in a percentage of consumers. One of the side effects engendered by vaccine ingredients is the production of IgE antibodies.[3] [4] The more effective a vaccine is, the greater the risks of allergies and other adverse effects.[5]

The question about vaccination has never been whether there would be damage but rather how much and what kind in relation to the established vaccination goals. Risk management for the five remaining vaccine manufacturers in the US was an ongoing concern. While the FDA had statutory responsibility for licensing vaccines, it appeared to lack the resources to fully grasp all safety issues. In 2004, researchers identified the need for an independent safety risk assessment system.[6] The system of post-licensure vaccine assessment was insufficient and hampered by perceived conflicts of interest.

Before 2000, doctors were beginning to admit that there was an uncomfortable unpredictability in combining different vaccine products in the same syringe.[7] [8] Doctors knew that iatrogenic conditions were being caused by vaccinations and yet, without comparative data on unvaccinated children officials were not compelled to reduce the pediatric schedule. In fact, it increased. The possibility of multiple vaccinations causing immune dysfunction was reviewed by the Institute of Medicine in 2002. The researchers admitted that they were unable to reach a satisfactory conclusion on the question. The primary obstacle to resolving the question was that they could not find research on an appropriate control group of unvaccinated children.[9] And the IOM had no authority to conduct its own scientific study.

In 2000 at a meeting of American adjuvant experts fatefully dubbed "Thimerosal 2",[10] doctors admitted that they did not know enough about the absorption, distribution and excretion of an adjuvant's aluminum from the body especially in infants. "Storage" of aluminum salts that can stimulate autoimmunity and allergy, was a problem for some children they agreed.[11]   Birth dose of aluminum, followed by regular doses of aluminum were excreted mostly by the kidneys although in a follow up study, 4% of the aluminum was still present over three years later.[12]   One of the meeting's speakers observed that somewhere in virtually every vaccinated child there remains a depot of the metal that the body does not want to release. Aluminum has an affinity for bone, kidney, brain and muscle.[13]

Another common vaccine ingredient is gelatin.   Gel is made from collagen derived from bovine or porcine hide and bones. It can also be made from tuna skin.[14]   In 1997, an outbreak of gelatin allergy in children startled doctors. Children were reacting to many foods that contained gelatin such as marshmallows, fruit gums, yoghurt and vitamin capsules.

In a rare admission, doctors confirmed that there was a causal link between the outbreak of gelatin allergy and the gelatin contained in a new diptheria-tetanus-acellular pertussis vaccine (DTaP).[15] [16]   Discontinuation of gelatin in this vaccine in 1999 reduced the prevalence of the allergy in children.[17]   However, gelatin continued to be used in other vaccines such as the MMR. Doctors admitted that this vaccine was also causing allergies to gelatin in children.[18] [19]

It was perhaps more difficult to conceive of peanut allergy in the same light. The idea that hundreds of thousands of children since the late 1980s had been made anaphylactic to peanut by some combination of vaccine ingredients was an incredible idea. And yet, few if any parents or family doctors were even aware that according to patent information many commonly used proprietary vaccine adjuvants contained refined peanut oil.[20]

The peanut oil label debate

As the peanut allergy epidemic spread, doctors and government expressed concern regarding the allergenicity of refined oil in processed foods and pharmaceuticals. They debated whether or not it should be labeled. Label reading had become something of a pastime for parents of allergic children. If any product listed peanut oil as an ingredient, refined or not, those parents would not purchase it. There were negative financial implications related to manufacturing with peanut oil.

At the same time, demand for the refined oil had increased in the manufacture of processed foods due to concerns over consumption of trans fats. Refined, bleached and deodorized (RBD) peanut oil was used in fried products, baked goods and as a flavor carrier.[21] It was considered a healthy alternative to other oils.

But the oil had been shown to cause both sensitization and reactions in a small number of people.[22] [23] The most highly refined peanut oils contain trace levels of intact proteins, up to $0.2\text{-}2.2\ \mu g/ml$.[24] [25] Lower quality refined peanut oils could contain $3\text{-}6\ \mu g/ml$ of protein. Thus, in 2004, the European Food Safety Authority (EFSA) investigated the safety of the oil and concluded that "fully refined peanut oil and fat" in foodstuffs could indeed cause allergic reactions in peanut allergic individuals.[26] The EFSA established a guideline that peanut oil must appear on food labels whether the oil is crude or refined.

In contrast, the WHO Codex Alimentarius Committee on Food Labeling in 2000 had expressed similar concerns but concluded that the oil in foodstuffs did not need to be labeled.[27] While this too was a guideline only, the fact that it was laid down by a panel of experts from around the world implied that it was reliable information. Laws would be made based on such guidelines.

The US FDA also acknowledged the presence of trace peanut proteins in the refined oil. However, they chose to grant the oil GRAS status (generally recognized as safe) since they believed no reactions had occurred from its consumption.[28] [29] In the US, it was not and is not mandatory to label refined peanut oil in foodstuffs.

But what of the peanut oil used in injectable drugs? Where the oil appeared as an excipient in parenteral drugs such as vaccines used in Europe the labeling arachis oil as of 2001 was required on package leaflets. It was expected that manufacturers should warn users that if one was allergic to peanut not to use this medicinal product.[30] These guidelines were produced by The Committee for Medicinal Products for Human Use (CHMP) at the European Medicines Agency (EMEA). The EMEA helps formulate vaccine package insert statements. Again, these were guidelines with an expectation of compliance and not laws. Deviations from the guidelines, according to the Agency, may be allowed if justified on a case-by-case basis. However, in the case of refined peanut oil, an agency representative confirmed that the consequences of ignoring the labeling guidelines could be serious. Allergic reactions to injected peanut oil in sensitive individuals can occur stated EMEA representative, George Wade:

> Patients have a right to know this information and it is also
> their right to have it presented to them in a clear, simple and
> unambiguous manner.[31]

In the US, labeling the oil in injected drugs remained voluntary. However, the FDA indicated that inactive ingredients that present an increased risk of toxic effects should be noted in the Contraindications, Warning or Precautions sections of drug labels.[32]

This labeling option in the US and Canada was supported by law. The exact composition of vaccines cannot and will not be disclosed under an exemption that protects business information within the Access to Information Act in Canada and the Freedom of Information Act in the US.

Similarly, trade secrets were also exempt under the British Freedom of Information Act.

The guidelines and the moral obligation to label peanut oil were in conflict with laws protecting trade secrets. Again, full disclosure of excipients that included adjuvants was not and continued not to be general practice in the US or Canada. Thus, labeling became a matter of least legal exposure within carefully worded vaccine product monographs. Whether parents were offered and read the monographs or not was another matter.

This labeling debate echoed concerns expressed in 1973 following the first media profiled peanut allergy death of a child. At the time, Dr. Jean Mayer, Professor of Nutrition at Harvard University wrote:

> We think food manufacturers should no more be allowed to hide behind "the need to protect recipe secrets" than drug manufacturers are. In both cases, lack of information can be not only unhealthy, but even deadly.[33]

Again, the facts that peanut proteins are so stable, resistant to digestive enzymes[34] and survive a rigorous refining process[35] would suggest that peanut oil was a poor choice for a vaccine additive intended to stimulate the immune system. Peanut is considered the perfect allergen.[36] [37]

Homology of peanut and Haemophilus type b (Hib)

Further complicating the outcome of vaccination was the apparent homology of the proteins of H. influenza b in the Hib vaccine and the proteins of peanut.

Homology simply refers to the similarity in the structure and the weight of protein molecules of different substances. Homology of molecules leads to cross reactivity. This phenomenon explains why a person allergic to peanut proteins may also react to nuts, even though they are from different plant families. The protein molecules of peanuts and those of tree nuts are homologous.[38]

The success of any vaccine design is in part built around the molecular weight(s) of the antigen. For example, studies indicate that protein conjugates made with low molecular weight dextran (polysaccharide) were more "immunogenic" than those made with dextrans of higher molecular weight.[39] In fact, molecules liable to bind more readily with blood serum are those with low molecular weight. Researchers have pointed to the low weight of drugs that must bind to carrier proteins in the body to elicit sensitization (less than 1,000 Da) whereas high molecular weight molecules (larger than 5,000 Da) can act as complete antigens and bind covalently on their own.[40]

It occurred to some researchers that Hib proteins, bound to their diphtheria or tetanus toxins or free floating and circulating in the blood stream, could result in an allergy to the Hib. Once sensitized to these proteins, there would exist the potential for cross reactivity to foods of homologous molecular weights: foods such as peanut.

The peanut protein Ara h 1 has a molecular weight of between 20 kDa and 63.5 kDa.[41] [42] A similar range exists for proteins of the Hib outer membrane – between 39 kDa[43] and 98 kDa.[44] Given this range, however, there would have been no practical way to confirm one way or the other whether there was the potential for cross reactivity.

The toxins used in the Hib vaccine were also cause for concern. In several allergy studies, mice were made allergic to peanuts by inhaling or eating the food mixed with a toxic bacterium. [45] It was possible that the toxins in the Hib vaccine – diphtheria and tetanus – had bonded with one of the most allergenic foods either in the vaccine oil excipient or extant in the human diet, peanuts.

Toxicity of Hib-DPT in creating peanut allergy

Anaphylaxis to the Hib vaccine including tetanus and diphtheria toxins it contained was surprisingly common. The natural bias of the infant immune system towards the Th2 response may have increased this allergic potential within an expanding and intense pediatric vaccination schedule.[46] [47] In fact, by 2000, anaphylaxis following vaccination had notably increased. Doctors admitted that this increase had "complicated" what used to be a routine procedure.[48]

Margie Profet elucidated the purpose of allergy in the vaccination event – whether the serum sickness of the early 20th century, postwar penicillin allergy or the massive rise in food allergy in children since 1990, the purpose of allergy is to protect the body against acute toxicity.[49]

Already it was well known that toxins from tetanus and diphtheria bacteria in the conjugate Hib vaccine frequently produced high levels of IgE and anaphylaxis in children. [50] [51] [52] [53] [54] [55] [56] [57] [58] [59] Indeed, bacterial toxins were well known adjuvants. It was possible, again, that these toxins which adjuvanted the Hib or other ingredients in the combined vaccines also enhanced the risk of cross reactivity to foods in the diet or food proteins in the vaccine.

A 1999 study hammered home this potential. It was found that pertussis bacteria had the ability to induce intestinal hypersensitivity and to prolong sensitization to foods in a mouse model. A mouse injected with ovalbumin showed IgE in jejunal segments that disappeared by 14 days. However, pertussis toxin with ovalbumin resulted in long-lasting sensitization present eight months after primary immunization. Bacteria when administered with a food protein resulted in long-term sensitization to the food and the antigen and altered intestinal immune function.[60]

In fact, medical literature was replete with examples of "how to" make an animal anaphylactic to foods by injecting it with toxic pathogens and peanut proteins. For example, mice were made anaphylactic to peanut through injections of heat-killed listeria and peanut,[61] a "cocktail" of measles vaccine and peanut,[62] and mycobacteria and peanut.[63] [64]

But when both Hib and its toxic conjugates were combined with a highly stimulating DPT vaccine, the immune response was even more pronounced. The Hib polysaccharide in a combination vaccine with DPT resulted in a more than 20-fold increase over the Hib alone.[65]

This over-stimulation of the immune system tipped the scales too far in favor of iatrogenic conditions including allergy.

Again the challenge in vaccine research was to gain potency while minimizing toxicity.[66] Many doctors saw toxicity and allergenicity as an acceptable compromise in the use of vaccine adjuvants. This compromise, for some doctors was an "accepted principle in the search for adjuvants suitable for use in human vaccines because one of their functions is to stimulate antigen presenting cells."[67]

Doctors seemed unaware, however, that the risk-benefit ratio had shifted.

The countries in which the peanut allergy first emerged were those that first paired the Hib with the DPT vaccine. Hib was not used in Russia, Japan, India, China, the Philippines, Romania, Korea, Iran, Singapore and other countries where peanut allergy was virtually unknown in 1997.

Singapore provided a poignant illustration of the impact of Hib-DPT combination when it was first introduced after 2001. In this country where full immunization of children was enforced by fine and imprisonment, Hib was optional, available for a fee. Since Hib was uncommon in Singaporean children doctors suggested that universal Hib vaccination program was not needed.[68] And yet, Singaporean parents had actually chosen and preferred to vaccinate with the convenient and combined acellular-pertussis-inactivated polio-Hib vaccine (DPTa-IPV/Hib).[69]

This combination had been approved for use in Singapore after 2001. At that time, sensitivity through skin prick tests to peanut showed that the allergy existed in Singapore but there were no reports of actual reactivity.[70] [71] By 2007, a three-year study revealed a "worrying trend" of peanut reactivity in Asian children living in Singapore (identifying with Chinese, Malay, Indian, and Eurasian ethnic groups).[72] Researchers there underscored the importance of examining environmental factors in this development but lack of exposure to peanuts was not one of them.

And doctors in Africa were puzzled by the high levels of IgE to peanut in children living in Ghana. Children there had received the five-in-one-shot containing DPT and Hib starting in 1992. In 2000, the Global Alliance for Vaccines and Immunization (GAVI) set a goal to fully vaccinate children under the age of one by 2010 in that country.[73] The hyporeactivity of the children was explained by the problematic prevalence of helminths. These parasitic worms depressed immune system reactivity.

But peanut allergy was virtually non-existent in western Siberia, Russia.[74] As of 2005, children were not vaccinated for Hib in Russia.[75]

And in India, where peanut allergy was also unknown, they have not vaccinated for Hib. However, a proposal to introduce the vaccine was made in 2008. Its proponents claimed it had become cost effective to do so.[76]

The Australian example

The history of changes to the pediatric schedules in Tasmania and the Australian Capital Territory provided yet another provocative illustration of the how and when peanut allergy emerged.

In a 2001 study, none of the 456 Tasmanian children aged 7–8 years reacted to a peanut skin-prick test.[77] By 2009, 1 in 90 children or 1.11%[78] were allergic to peanuts. Changes in the vaccination schedule and the increased rate of children vaccinated in Tasmania correlated to this development.

In 1997, Tasmanian children were the least likely to be vaccinated at 27% of children according to the Australian Bureau of Statistics.[79] Vaccination rates were dramatically low and declining on this island of about 500,000 people. In 1998, only 21% of children were vaccinated by their first year.[80]

In 1998, the Australian government established a General Practice Immunization Initiative that intensified the pediatric schedule and national coverage for preschool children including those in Tasmania. The goal was to have over 90% of the children vaccinated. In 2001, the Australian government implemented their strategy[81] [82] [83] and surpassed their goal by vaccinating 94% of Tasmanian children by age one. Tasmania became the highest vaccinated population in the country.[84] By 2009, 1.11% of Tasmanian children were allergic to peanuts.

In contrast to the sudden growth of the allergy in Tasmanian, peanut allergy in children living in the Australian Capital Territory (ACT)[85] grew steadily. By 1995, .5% of ACT children were peanut allergic. [86] By 2001, .71% of ACT children were allergic and by 2009 2% of "school entrant" ACT children were confirmed as peanut allergic.[87] Children living in this national political centre were the most likely to be fully immunized at 48% in 1995[88] according to the Australian Bureau of Statistics. Changes to the pediatric schedule of ACT were similar to but made less rapidly than those in the US and the UK. The changes to the schedules for ACT and Tasmania were, of course, the same. But again, the primary difference between Tasmanian children and those living in ACT was vast differences in rate of vaccination. Government programs attempted to harmonize this rate in 2001.

Idiosyncrasies

But if the pediatric vaccination schedule was causing peanut allergy, why were all children not allergic? Why, even in the same family, was one vaccinated child peanut allergic and another one was not?

Allergy is designed to defend against toxins that escape general detoxification. This being true, the potential for allergic sensitization to drugs and the ability to detoxify those drugs are inversely related, suggested Profet.[89] The ability of peanut allergic children to eliminate toxins including those from the vaccines was challenged at the time of vaccination.

Bock pointed to four catastrophic changes that have contributed to the rise of allergy as well as asthma, autism and ADHD: toxins have proliferated; nutrition has deteriorated; vaccinations have increased; children's abilities to detoxify have dwindled. Methylation and sulfation, two important detoxification processes responsible for removing mercury and other toxins have been damaged, suggested Bock.[90]

Children with severe allergy exhibit an immune system overload[91] caused by: antibiotic overuse; fungal overgrowth; overactivitiy of the Th2 cells; and childhood vaccinations. The fungal infection that began in the gut was made worse by poor eating habits and deficiencies in: nutrition; probiotics; essential fatty acids; stomach acid; and digestive enzymes. Further challenging the child was maternal health. Fungal infection was passed to unborn children. Birth by cesarean that delayed the introduction of healthy digestive flora would only have exacerbated the condition.

Gender also played an enormous role in who developed the peanut allergy. The allergy appeared more often in boys than girls – the ratio greater than 2:1.[92 93 94 95] A male predominance of peanut and tree nut allergy was reported in children younger than 18 years – 1.7% vs. 0.7% males to females.[96]

While there was no clear explanation for this disparity, a parallel phenomenon had occurred in the prevalence of autism where boys were affected more than girls in a 4:1 ratio.

This gender gap was as high as 10:1 for Asperger's Syndrome. In 1964, Bernard Rimland observed that boys tended to be more vulnerable to "organic damage" than girls whether through hereditary disease, acquired infection or other conditions.

The rate of autism and peanut allergy in children increased within the same window of time starting around 1990 with a concomitant sex ratio difference. The rate of autism in the US was believed to be 1 in 1,000 in 1970.[97] In 2009, it was more than 1 in 100 children in the US. Peanut allergy had no significant profile prior to 1990. In 2009, about 2% of children were allergic to peanuts.

And so, children with an extant immune overload caused by various deficiencies, fungal infection and impaired detoxification processes responded adversely to the new and intense vaccination schedule launched around 1990.

Screening children before vaccination would have been a way to reduce risks but was not common practice before the terrific increase in allergies that occurred. Even with the few questions posed to parents in 2009 prior to vaccination, no inquiry was made into the child's sulfation and methylation processes, kidney health, mitochondrial function or whether mother and child had fungal infections.

A vetting process based on idiosyncrasy was antithetical to the aims of mass and routine vaccination. A thorough screening would also challenge the cost effectiveness of vaccination. Vaccination was alleged to save money otherwise lost should working parents have to stay home to care for their sick children. This affected the national economy. And if many children were found to be at high risk of adverse reaction, they would have to be exempted from vaccination. How would society manage this scenario?

Conversely, what was the financial cost of peanut allergy to society? Since the parents and allergic children absorbed the damage there was little or no financial burden on government or society although it challenged the peanut industry. Peanut allergy families coped through avoidance strategies and school communities modified their behavior to accommodate the growing problem. Alternatively, revenues were being generated through peanut and other food allergic children in the US – more than three million children in 2008 – fueled a burgeoning Food Allergy Industry through the purchase of drugs and free-from foods.

Chapter 7

Rationalizations

The crossover point

In 2009, there was a 1 in 50 chance that a child, especially a male living in the US, Canada, the UK, Australia, Sweden and a handful of other western countries would develop the peanut allergy. When asked what was causing this epidemic, doctors deferred to the Hygiene Hypothesis or simply stated that they did not know.

And yet, medical literature illustrated that the only means by which mass allergy had ever been created was by injection. With the pairing of the hypodermic needle and vaccine at the close of the 19th century, allergy and anaphylaxis made their explosive entry into the western world. Serum sickness from this new procedure was the first mass allergic phenomenon in history. Epidemic allergy to penicillin reminiscent of the "days of serum sickness" emerged with its mass application following WW II. And with it came peanut allergy. Penicillin was administered using POB, the Romansky peanut oil formula. The continued use of refined peanut oil in drugs and vaccine adjuvants resulted in the slow growth of the allergy primarily in children until the late 1980s when its prevalence exploded. Extensive and sudden changes to childhood vaccinations precipitated the new mass allergy to peanut.

Whether the smoking gun was a cross-reactive Hib protein, peanut oil, adjuvants and toxins within the novel five-vaccines-in-one shot, it made little difference. There were so few candidates of functional causation that could touch just children and just in the west that by its very absence from the plethora of research on the peanut allergy, injection was the most obvious suspect. One could not argue with ER records, eyewitness accounts and cohort studies that all pointed to a specific moment around 1990, when peanut and other food allergies in children suddenly escalated.

What could have had the power to create an allergy in hundreds of thousands of western children at the same time in history to the same food? Clearly, there was a functional mechanism for this mass sensitization. Coincidence, digestive failure, peanut oil skin creams or genetics could not explain it.

Doctors knew that as the number and potency of vaccines increased, so too would the risk of side effects that included soaring IgE and atopy.[1] Anaphylaxis immediately following vaccination had finally become an "obstacle" to the routine jab, doctors observed.[2] But any suspicion that peanut allergy was being caused by vaccination, however, was quickly trapped within a complex weave of conflicting agendas held by government, medical authorities, pharmaceutical corporations and the media.

At stake in any hint of culpability were the reputations and incomes of doctors and scientists, the interests and power of medical associations, corporate revenues, shareholders interests, the authority of government and its control over the health of entire populations.[3] It was a rare doctor who stepped outside of this awesome mesh to wonder in print whether multiple vaccines were worth the massive rise in atopy.[4]

There were several rational arguments doctors used for not publicly pursuing the connection between the new expanded schedule imposed on children starting in the late 1980s and the rise in peanut allergy.

The first rationalization was that Vaccine Injury Compensation Program guidelines in the US made it impossible to prove a causal link between vaccination and a later "onset" of a life-threatening allergy – that is, in the case of peanut allergy, when the toddler first eats and reacts to peanut butter months after vaccination. The guidelines only recognized damage that occurred shortly after injection.

Richet himself who wrote that anaphylaxis "perhaps a sorry matter for the individual, is necessary to the species" summarized the second rationalization. "There is something more important than the salvation of the person and that is integral preservation of the race."[5] The aim of protecting the whole of society from disease through vaccination of children justified the unavoidable casualties.

The third rationalization was economic. Vaccine consumers absorbed the costs of damage. Therefore, it made financial sense on the part of the pharmaceutical companies and governments to ignore the problem – which could not be proven anyway. The IOM admitted that they were unable to analyze and, therefore, deduce a connection between allergic conditions in children and vaccination because there were no acceptable unvaccinated populations in the US. There was no control group. Amish communities in which peanut allergy was virtually unknown also discourage vaccination. However, because these communities were genetically linked their example was inadmissible.

And finally, if sympathetic courts allowed litigation from concerned parents, government would intercede with legislation to control it as it did in 1986 with the National Childhood Vaccine Injury Act. This Act provided a no-fault alternative to the tort system in which the federal government cushioned the relationship between the public and the pharmaceutical companies with new rules and money.

The way individuals experienced risk in society had changed substantially since the days of Jenner or Pasteur. In the early days of vaccination, a social contract of sorts was forged between populations and the medical community that assured people of better odds if they were vaccinated. This may have been proven right in many cases, but the risks were in the open and if you were frightened enough you had the vaccination – mandatory vaccination laws, disease mongering and scare tactics helped you make a decision but the risks were evident. As the century unfolded, risks associated with vaccination were delineated for the public by government, politicians and medical authorities via the mass media.

Parents were assuaged by the institutional language of medical officials who explained that "routine immunizations do not increase the risk of babies developing allergic disorders and are safe to give to babies with food allergies, eczema, or asthma".[6] In truth, parents were hard pressed to know what they were actually doing when they vaccinated their children. Even vaccine labels did not disclose complete ingredients. As ever, parents relied on doctors to explain the procedure perhaps not realizing that in the event of an adverse reaction, they and their child would be abandoned by the system they trusted and branded criminals should they stop vaccinating.

The landmark non-fiction horror *A Shot in the Dark* (1991) written by a medical researcher and an angry mother forced many to think about vaccination from the consumer's perspective. Their book highlighted the degree to which medical authorities and government had shifted responsibility for vaccine damage away from pharmaceutical companies and doctors by placing onus for proof on parents.

Helping parents understand the role of vaccination in the dramatic rise of autism in US children became a cause for parents like celebrity Jenny McCarthy. McCarthy's non-profit organization Generation Rescue launched a vaccine awareness campaign in 2005. The *Green Our Vaccines* campaign asked, "Why are we giving our children so many more vaccines so early in life?" US children receive their first shot within hours of birth and a total of 36 different vaccines in their first two years. In 1970, when children received about 10 vaccines, the rate of autism in the US was about 1 in 1,000. In 2008, the rate was 1 in 150. In 2009, new reports suggested that number was about 1 in 100.

The epidemic rise of autism parallels that of the peanut allergy – in the period of its acceleration and gender bias. Many autistic children also have severe food allergies. When a link was made between vaccination and autism, the US government, vaccine makers and the media attempted to squash it. The manner in which this issue was addressed offers a glimpse into the future of the peanut allergy.

In 2000, a confidential report *Thimerosal VSD Study, Phase I* (2000) from the CDC linked the rise in autism to a mercury based anti-fungal vaccine ingredient, Thimerosal. The Eli Lilly Co., a company founded by Civil War veteran Eli Lilly, developed Thimerosal in the 1930s. An emergency meeting held at the Simpsonwood Retreat Center in Georgia was called by the CDC and attended by 52 vaccine experts and pharmaceutical company representatives. A transcript of the meeting leaked to the Internet revealed how frightened doctors were by this government revelation. Here was the basis for ruinous class action lawsuits and serious loss of public confidence in vaccination.

While the Thimerosal report ultimately was made available, its original supporting data was lost. At the same time, the database of approximately 100,000 children on which the report was based was given to a private company beyond the reach of the Freedom of Information Act.

In 2000, the maker of Thimerosal, Eli Lilly Co. was shielded from prosecution by parents of autistic children when House Majority Leader Dick Armey put the "Eli Lilly Protection Act" into the Homeland Security Act.[7] [8]

When this Act was repealed in 2003, US Senate Majority Leader Bill Frist in 2008 added a provision to an anti-terrorism bill that denied compensation to children suffering from vaccine related brain disorders. In a post 9-11 world, Frist explained, US companies needed protection from cumbersome and costly lawsuits so that they were free to produce vaccines in the event of a bio-terrorist attack.[9]

Despite government assurance that Thimerosal would be phased out of childhood vaccines, doing so would prove difficult. One doctor at the Simpsonwood meeting announced:

> My mandate as I sit here in this group is to make sure at the end of the day that 100,000,000 are immunized with DPT, Hepatitis B and if possible Hib, this year, next year and for many years come, and that will have to be with Thimerosal containing vaccines unless a miracle occurs and an alternative is found quickly and is tried and found to be safe.[10]

The doctor's urgent hyperbole revealed much about the two-day meeting; there were just 19 million children under five years of age in 2000.

The public was led to believe that Thimerosal had been removed from the pediatric schedule. A statement to this effect was produced by the California Dept. of Developmental Services and supported by the American Academy of Family Physicians. In the same statement, however, the state government admitted that trace levels existed in all vaccines and that some childhood vaccines contained original levels. They did not indicate which ones. It seemed, then, that all childhood vaccines in 2009 still contained Thimerosal, to one degree or another.[11]

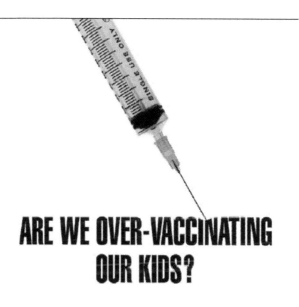

The *Green Vaccine Campaign* was launched by Generation Rescue, a non-profit organization in California dedicated to the support of autistic children and their families.

Since the rate of autism continued to rise despite the erroneous ˊclaim that the Thimerosal was gone, the media attempted to close the case. A *Time Magazine* article gave the "truth" about vaccination accusing all parents who questioned it of putting "the rest of us at risk".[12] The simplistic "us vs. them" fiction boiled the discussion down into an easy to understand concept of personal belief vs. public health. This tactic successfully drew attention away from the seminal issue of disease management and adverse events to target and ostracize a new, fictitious enemy - concerned parents who believed their children had been damaged by injections.

No longer patients or even medical consumers, the parents who chose not to vaccinate were painted as dangerous and criminally minded people. Some determined Americans, however, fought back. In 2009, a media driven influenza scare led to federally mandated flu shots that trampled constitutional rights. Concerned citizens were forced to sue their government. A preliminary injunction to halt federal mandatory flu vaccinations in the state of New Jersey was issued in August, 2009.[13] [14]

The "us vs. them" dialectic also drew attention away from the money. Vaccination was less about medicine than it was about economics. Pharmaceutical company CEOs must, by law, protect their shareholders first. If there was damage, they would not and could not admit it unless it was in the best interest of their company. Case in point, one pharmaceutical company CEO quoted in a 2006 article, reflected that the problem with most adjuvanted vaccines was that their potency caused allergies. While his company's brand was not as potent as others, it was safer.[15] This unusually frank disclosure was used to sell his company's products and enhance shareholder value.

Government mass vaccinates populations to protect the economy. In deciding, for example, which diseases needed to be addressed first through vaccination, the

IOM in 1985 applied an economic model that included the anticipated net savings of health care resources. In 2003, the economic burden of influenza in the US was an estimated $87.1 Billion including direct medical costs and indirect costs to employers and lost productivity.[16]

This cost-effective justification does not work for the Hib vaccine, however. In comparing the treatment costs averted by a theoretical burden of Hib and cost of vaccine application, a 2005 article supposed that vaccination would reduce direct disease costs by $18 Million and decrease productive losses by $50 Million.[17] WHO publications described the Hib vaccine as a "blockbuster" product.[18] The vaccine market in 1998 was an estimated $5.4 Billion and was expected to increase by 12% a year. The revenues generated by sales of the vaccine were enormous compared to the theoretical savings in this instance. A significant portion of this became pharmaceutical revenues.

In 2006, the pharmaceutical industry profits increased $8 Billion in the six-month period following the start of the new US Medicare drug program in Jan. 1, 2006. Profit in 2006 in just six months for the top 10 makers was $39,780,689,350.[19]

In addition to theoretical cost savings for government and corporate profits there were concrete cost downloads to consumers. The costs of vaccine damage such as allergy was not built into the government model of disease management because they were absorbed by those affected – children and their parents. These people in turn have spawned a new source of revenue for business. The rise in food allergy and intolerance has contributed to an enormous free-from food market. The market for gluten free, lactose free, peanut free, sugar free and other free from foods was an estimated $3.9 Billion in 2008.[20]

The massive rise in chronic degenerative conditions in children has made money for investors in pharmaceutical stocks, as well. One market analyst suggested that given the explosion in allergy in children that an "Autoimmune Index" would be a useful tool for investors. This Index would help them choose profitable pharmaceutical stocks relative to the rise in such childhood epidemics as peanut allergy, Crohn's, MS, and diabetes.[21]

Was it more profitable then to continue producing allergy than it was to change vaccination schedules and screen children to prevent the allergy in the first place?

And what of the role of parents in making and supporting the tradition of mass vaccination? Society as a whole must share the responsiblility for producing the epidemic.

Shaw opined in the Preface to the *Doctor's Dilemma* (1909), "Until there is a practicable alternative to blind trust in the doctor, the truth about the doctor is so terrible that we dare not face it." Yet by 2009, 100 years after Shaw's vitriol and the first decades of the tradition of mass vaccination, the balance between fear of disease and the risk of side effects had shifted. Medical consumers especially parents of the millions of children with autism and anaphylaxis have or are developing a new appreciation for the risks related to vaccinations.

This change in public tolerance was a red flag to Stanford University School of Medicine Dr. Eugene Robin.[22] This elderly doctor pointed to the shifting of the ratio in the number of cases of a given disease to the complications caused by the vaccine. It was a process he called the "crossover point" where the complication rate of a vaccine for individuals becomes higher than the adverse effects of the disease.

Robin asked readers including government and pharmaceutical companies to consider a scenario in which a highly effective vaccine over time progressively decreases the incidence of the disease. When the percentage of adverse events associated with the vaccine remained constant or even increased as the disease became less threatening, society will have reached the crossover point. At that point, wrote Robin, the wise thing for uncomfortable parents to do would be to refuse vaccination.

Parents of autistic children reached the crossover point in 2000 – bands of parents in the US became organized, well informed and militant. They refused to live with this condition and were determined to help other parents prevent it in their children.

Parents of peanut allergic children, however, were coping. But as the epidemic prevalence of peanut and other life threatening food allergies in children spread, these parents too began to take a stand.

Appendix

Using that modest percentage 1.04% in 2003 for the top five peanut allergy countries, the total pediatric peanut allergic population was greater than 4.3 million. This number is believed to have doubled to approximately 8 million with the peanut allergic children growing into an adult statistic. The following figures reveal an upward trend for affected countries.

AFRICA

- In Ghana, serologic evidence of peanut sensitivity was found in about 2% school children between 5 and 16 years of age (2009).[1] .53% of children in this study had an "adverse reaction" to peanut. Top food allergens were pineapple and peanut. Serologic evidence of sensitivity in 5% of Xhosan children in Cape Town (2007)[2] but with no reported cases of anaphylaxis.

SUB-SARHARA, NORTH AFRICA

- 0% Sub-Sahara (2006) – Prof. Gideon Lack, in a speech, noted in the *British Medical Journal* the absence of peanut allergy in this part of the world; peanuts are a staple for children at weaning and beyond.[3]

AUSTRALIAN CAPITAL TERRITORY (ACT), AUSTRALIA

- 2% (2009) of school entrant ACT children were confirmed by diagnostic test to be peanut allergic.[4] ACT is a self-governing state with the highest density population and smallest area at 2,358 km[2]. Within it is the national capital of Canberra. According to the Australasian Society of Clinical Immunology and Allergy, 1.15% of ACT children born in 2004 were peanut allergic. Compared to .47% of those born in 1995.[5] National figures for Australia are: .71% (2001),[6] .5% (1995).[7] Children make up 26% of the Australian population. Therefore, in 2009 of almost 22 million Australians there were about 5.7 million children with 114,400 of them peanut allergic.

TASMANIA, AUSTRALIA

- 1.11% (2009)[8], 0% (2001)[9]. Of a population-based cohort of 456 Tasmanian children aged 7–8 years, none reacted to a peanut skin-prick test in 2001. By 2009, 1.11% of children were reactive to peanut.

MONTREAL, CANADA

- 1.71+% of children under 9 in Montreal, Canada (2007). [10] [11] In 2009 there were 7.8534 million children in Canada under 19. Therefore, 134,293 children were peanut allergic.

NORTH-EASTERN EUROPE

- Geographically close countries in North Eastern Europe – Estonia, Lithuania and Russia – appear to have a very low prevalence of peanut allergy.[12]

FRANCE

- .45+% of children under 15 in France (2002) were peanut allergic.[13] [14]

GERMANY

- No firm statistics are available although peanut allergy seems of limited significance. In a 2005 analysis of physician reported cases of 103 anaphylactic children in Germany, foods were the most frequent cause of the reaction (57%, and of this number 20% to peanut) followed by insect stings (13%) and immunotherapy injections (12%). Peanuts and tree nuts were the foods most frequently causing the reactions.[15] In a 2004 study of food allergy in Berlin children and teens, there appeared to be no self-reported symptoms to peanut.[16]

HONG KONG

- .57% to 1% of Chinese children aged 2 – 7 living in Hong Kong[17] were reactive to peanut (2009). A Europrevall Prague report indicated that .7% of Hong Kong study participants were peanut allergic (2008). Studies published in 1994[18] and 1999[19], concluded that sensitization to peanut was rare in Chinese children living in Hong Kong. In fact, it seemed rare to find peanut allergy at all in South-East Asia.[20] Subsequent reports 2001/2002 re-iterated that while the per capita consumption of peanuts in China is similar to that of the US, peanut allergy was rare in China. By 2008, .57 to 1% of Chinese children were reacting to peanut. Chinese-American children living in the US had an incidence of peanut allergy similar to that of the general US population (2001).[21]

INDIA

- No apparent studies of peanut allergy have come from India. Peanuts are cheap sources of dietary protein in India and are called the "poor man's nut". They are the chief ingredient of baby food products introduced to children as early as six months of age. Peanut allergy is not known in this part of the world or possibly the symptoms of the reaction (if any) are not attributed to peanut.[22]

ISRAEL

- 0.17% of children (2006) in Israel react to peanuts.[23] Researchers found that UK children had a prevalence of peanut allergy that was 10-fold higher than that of children from Israel – 1.85% versus 0.17 percent.[24] However, sesame is the equivalent of peanut allergy in Israel. It is the 2nd most common food allergy in toddlers after cow's milk, and is less likely to resolve.[25] The sesame allergy epidemic in Israel is a mystery.

. JAPAN

- In 2003, population-based prevalence figures for food allergy in Japan were apparently unavailable.[26] The most common food allergen among Japanese children was hen's egg, followed by cow's milk and wheat. These three food allergens accounted for 60% of pediatric food allergy. Foods with increasing frequency of allergic reactions among children were peanuts, sesame, and fruit.

NORWAY, DENMARK

- 0.5% in Danish adolescents in 2005 reacted to peanuts.[27] In 2001, the numbers of peanut allergic children in Norway, Denmark were believed to be very low.[28]

SINGAPORE

- 1.08% – 1.35% of children aged 5 to 12 living in Singapore were reactive to peanut in 2007.[29] A 1997 study had alluded to reports of peanut allergy from several Asian centers including Singapore, Philippines, Malaysia, Indonesia, Japan, Beijing, Hong Kong and Taiwan.[30] Sensitization to peanut was second to shellfish in cohort under 5 according to a National University of Singapore professor (2005). Significantly, although children were sensitized to peanut there were no reported cases of anaphylaxis. The reason for this was not known although lack of exposure to peanuts was not a factor.[31] However, by 2007, a three-year study revealed a "worrying trend" of peanut reactivity in Asian children living in Singapore (Chinese, Malay, Indian and Eurasian ethnic groups).[32] Peanut allergy was found in 27.3% of food allergic children.

SWEDEN

- 1.2+% of children under 6 in Sweden (1998) were reactive to peanut.[33] [34] In 2000, 2.139 million people were under age 19. Therefore, 25,668 children were allergic to peanuts in 1998.

UK

- 2+% of infants and young children were allergic to peanuts in 2009.[35] In 2008 there were 11.5 million children under 16. Therefore, an estimated 230,000 children in the UK were allergic to peanut. Another statistic indicated that 1 in 70 children (1.43%) were allergic to peanut.[36] [37] [38]

US

- 1.2+% children under 18 (2002) were reactive to peanut. [39] [40] [41] [42] [43] [44] In 2002, there were 871,200 peanut allergic children (72.6 million children under 18 in 2002). In 2009 this number have been as high as 1.45 million.

171

End Notes

The Problem of the Peanut Allergy

1 See Appendix.

2 The World Health Organization's Codex Alimentarius Commission (est. 1963) created a list of critical food allergens in 1996: peanut, tree nut, fish, shellfish, wheat, soy, dairy, egg. These eight account for about 90% of all food reactions.

3 The peanut epitopes are: Ara h 1; Ara h2 (5 subtypes); Ara h3 through 8; Ara h Agglutinin; Ara h LTP; Ara h Oleosin; Ara h T1.

4 R. Fischer, et al., "Oral and nasal sensitization promote distinct Immune responses and lung reactivity in mouse model of peanut allergy," *Am J Pathol.*, 16, 6 (Dec., 2005): 1621-1630; C.A. Coop, et al., "Anaphylaxis from the influenza virus vaccine," *Int Arch Allergy Immunol.*, 146, 1 (2008): 85-8.

5 Margie Profet, "The Function of Allergy: Immunological defense against toxins", *The Quarterly Review of Biology*, 66, 1 (March, 1991): 23-62.

6 H. Zinsser, T. Tamiya, "An experimental analysis of bacterial allergy," *The Journal of Experimental Medicine*, 44 (1926): 753-776.

7 V.I. Klots, "The case of allergy to cholera vaccine," *Foreign Technology Division Wright Patterson AFB, Ohio, Defense Technical Information Center* (Oct. 9, 1974). http://oai.dtic.mil/oai/oai?verb=getRecord&metadataPrefix=html&identifier=ADA000172

8 M. Modrzynski, et al., "The occurrence of food allergy and bacterial allergy n children with tonsilar hypertrophy," *Przegl Lek*, 61,12 (2004):1330-3.

9 C.J. Hackett, D.A. Ham (ed.), *Vaccine adjuvants: immunological and clinical principals* (Humana Press, 2006) 139.

10 Klaus Erb, "Can helminths or helminth-derived products be used in humans to prevent or treat allergic diseases?" *Trends in Immunology*, 30, 2 (Feb. 2009): 75-82.

11 Profet, Op. cit.

12 I.N. Glaspole, et al., "Anaphylaxis to lemon soap: citrus seed and peanut allergen cross-reactivity," *Ann Allergy Asthma Immunol.*, 98, 3 (March, 2007): 286-9.

13 Quoted in Alice Park, "The Truth About Vaccines," *Time Magazine* (Canadian Edition, June 2, 2008) 34.

14 M.R. Odent, "Long term effects of early vaccinations," *Primal Health Research Newsletter*, 2, 1 (1994): 6.

15 G.W. Ewing, "What is regressive autism and why does it occur? Is it the consequence of multi-system dysfunction affecting the elimination of heavy metals and the ability to regulate neural temperature?" *North American Journal of Medical Sciences*, 1, 2 (July, 2009): 34. See also A.W. Taylor-Robinson, "Multiple vaccination effects on atopy," *Allergy*, 54 (April, 1999): 398-399.

16 H. Albonico, et al., "The immunization campaign against measles, mumps and rubella – coercion leading to a realm of uncertainty: medical objections to a continued MMR immunization campaign in Switzerland," *JAMA*, 9, 1 (1992).

17 James Altucher, "Save the children (and make money)," *The Wall Street Journal* (August 10, 2009). http://online.wsj.com/article/SB124992390387319939.html

CHAPTER 1: From Idiosyncrasy to Multi-Billion Dollar Industry

1 Anon, "Doctor nearly dies of salted peanuts," *The New York Times, Books Section*, (Mon., Dec. 20, 1954) 31.

2 Perhaps the very first documented nut allergy was a case study in 1920 by noted hematologist Dr. Kenneth Blackfan in England. The doctor observed a 10-year-old child, whose eczema was "intensified" by nuts, eggs and fish.

3 George W. Gray, "Allergy, protection gone wild," *Harper's Magazine* rerun in the *Milwaukee Journal* (Sat., Jan. 1, 1939).

4 Anon, "Doctor finds a new drug to treat allergies," *Chicago Tribune* (April 17, 1949).

5 *Allergy to Cottonseed and Other Oilseeds and their Edible Derivatives. Excerpts from Testimony before the Administrator, Federal Security Agency, in the matter of fixing and establishing definitions and standards of identity for mayonnaise, French dressing, and related salad dressings* (US Federal Security Agency and the National Cottonseed Products Association, 1948). This book documents public hearings held in Washington (Nov. 1947 - Jan., 1948) in which doctors and cottonseed oil workers testified on the safety of refined cottonseed oil and lack of standards in the crushing industry which led to cross contamination of many oils subsequently used in various processed foods. Articles on "hypersensitivity" and allergy to cottonseed appeared in 1940s and 50s in *Pediatrics, Annals of Allergy, Journal of American Medical Association, Acta allergologica.*

6 Cottonseed allergy and anaphylaxis were reported in Judy E. Perkin (ed.), *Food allergies and adverse reactions* (Aspen, 1990) 57. Cottonseed oil is used in medications and foods including mayonnaise, fried potato chips, oil packed tuna. Cottonseed flour may be found in baked goods, candy, spices, cream substitutes and processed meats.

7 G. Hildick-Smith, et al., "Penicillin Regimens in Pediatric Practice: Study of Blood Levels," *Pediatrics* (Jan. 1950): 97-113. This article reports that the Romansky Formula created sensitivity to peanut oil in a study of children at the Children's Hospital of Philadelphia. See also P.C. Trussell et al., "Duration of Effective Blood levels following administration of penicillin in peanut oil and beeswax," *Canad. M.A.J.*, 57 (Oct. 1947): 387; R.V. Platou, et al., "Round Table Discussion on Antibiotics," *Pediatrics* (Feb. 1948).

8 A.P. Black, "A new diagnostic method in allergic disease," *Pediatrics*, 17 (May, 1956): 716-724; S. Goldman, et al, "Milk Allergy," *Pediatrics*, 32 (Sept. 1963): 425-443; and W.G. Crook, et al, "Systemic Manifestations due to allergy: Report on Fifty Patients," Pediatrics, 27 (May, 1961): 790-799. Both articles observe an increase in peanut and food allergy in children.

9 Jean Mayer, "Better labeling laws are needed," *Pittsburgh Post-Gazette* (June 5, 1972) 12.

10 S.A. Bock, F.M. Atkins, "The natural history of peanut allergy*" The Journal of allergy and Clinical Immunology*, 83, 5 (June 1, 1989): 900-4. Bock and others pioneered the use of the double blind placebo controlled food challenge (DBPCFC).

11 F. Speer, "Multiple food allergy," *Ann Allergy*, 34, 2 (Feb., 1975): 71-6. Further studies indicated that peanut allergic children typically had multiple food allergies.

12 http://www.sarnoffendowment.org/about/history.cfm

13 Anon, "Candy kills peanut allergic youth," *The Spokesman-Review, Washington* (Sept. 28, 1980).

14 Anon (UPI), "Allergy kills Brown student," *New York Times* (June 5, 1986).

15 Anon, "Stricken in the cabin," *LA Times* (April 1, 1988).

16 Warren Vaughan, *Strange Malady, The Story of Allergy* (New York: Doubleday, Doran & Co., 1941) 111.

17 Anon, "Bite of cake ends a boy's struggle for life," *Sacramento Bean and Gainsville Sun* (Jan. 16, 1987); "Allergic reaction death," *Ocala Star-Banner* (Jan. 16, 1987); "When food becomes poison," *The Ledger* (Sept. 10, 1987); "A lot of food hazard hides in undercooked vittles," *The Courier* (Oct. 28, 1987) "...every week brings reports of new dangers; a death from allergy..."

18 Anon, "How to prevent severe allergic reactions," *St. Petersburg Times* (July 21, 1988); "Those with deadly allergies need epinephrine," *The Ledger* (July 21, 1988); "Many treatments available for hives," *Chicago Tribune* (July 29, 1988); "Battling deadly allergies, stimulant epinephrine can help victims," *St. Petersburg Times* (July 21, 1988); "Allergy-prone people advised on fast relief in simple kit," *LA Times* (July 24, 1988); "People with potentially deadly allergies require epinephrine," *Ludington Daily News* (Sept. 9, 1988).

19 Anon, "When your immune system panics, anaphylaxis, severe allergic reaction," *The Saturday Evening Post* (Oct. 1, 1989); "Listing ingredients for allergy sufferers," *St. Louis Post-Dispatch* (Jan. 9, 1989) reflects on 1986 peanut-chili death; "Children at risk from things safe for adults," *Daily News of LA* (April 3, 1989); "Body and mind: backward protection," *NY Times* (July 2, 1989); "Allergy guide makes shopping for special foods easier," *The Gazette, Colorado Springs* (Feb. 15, 1989)

20 Anon, "Food allergies: cause for concern or over-diagnosed malady?" *Environmental Nutrition* (Nov. 1, 1989).

21 S. A. Bock, et al, "Fatalities due to anaphylactic reactions to food," *Journal of Allergy and Clinical Immun.*, 107, 1 (Jan., 2001): 191-93.

22 A.M. Barnam, S.L. Lukacs, "Food allergy among U.S. children: trends in prevalence and hospitalizations," National Centre for Health Statistics, CDC (Oct. 22, 2008). This trend continued. Four in every 100 US children in 2008 had a severe food allergy.

23 R.J. Mullins, "Paediatric food allergy trends in a community-based specialist allergy practice, 1995-2006," *Medical Journal of Australia*, 186,12 (2007): 618-621.

24 A. Sheik, "Life threatening allergy, an homage to Von Pirquet," *World Allergy Forum Symposium* (Sun. June 11, 2006). Lecture recorded in Vienna, Austria http://www.worldallergy.org/educational_programs/world_allergy_forum/vienna2006/syllabus_book.pdf; R. Gupta, A. Sheikh, et al. "Increasing hospital admissions for systemic allergic disorders in England: analysis of national admissions data," *BMJ*, 327 (Nov., 2003): 1142-1143.

25 http://www.foodnavigator.com/Science-Nutrition/Peanut-allergies-rising-reveals-UK-study

26 J. Grundy, et al., "Rising prevalence of allergy to peanut in children: data from 2 sequential cohorts," *Journal of Allergy and Clinical Immunology*, 110, 5 (Nov. 2002).

27 Anon, "Parents warned of peanut risk to children," *The Independent* (April 26, 1996); "40,000 children in peril from peanuts; the growing taste that can kill," *The Mirror* (April 2, 1996).

28 http://www.foodnavigator.com/Science-Nutrition/Peanut-allergies-rising-reveals-UK-study

29 J. Grundy, Op. cit.

30 C. Thompson, "One bite and he dies", *Sunday Times Magazine* (19 Oct. 1997) 24-8; S. de Bruxelles, "Nuts led to death of allergic scientist", *The Times* (Nov. 21, 1997); T. Burchill, "The rise of killer food", *The Times*, T2 (Jan. 22, 2002) 10; D. Hide, "Fatal anaphylaxis due to food," *BMJ*, 307 (27 Nov. 27, 1993): 1427; E.S.K. Assem, et al, "Anaphylaxis induced by peanuts", *BMJ*, 307 (May 26, 1990): 1377.

31 L. Chiu, et al. "Estimation of the sensitization rate to peanut by prick skin test in the general population: results from the National Health and Nutrition Examination Survey, 1980-1994," *J Allergy Clin Immunol.*, 107 (2001): S192.

32 K. Beyer, et al., "Effects of cooking methods on peanut allergenicity," *Journal of Allergy and Clinical Immunology*, 107, 6 (June 2001): 1077-1081.

33 S.A. Bock, et al., "Fatalities due to anaphylactic reactions to foods," *J. Allergy Clin. Immunol.*,107 (2001): 191-193.

34 Anon, "Experiment produces promising allergy therapy injections ease reaction to peanuts," *Charlotte Observer* (March 12, 1992).

35 A. Gosline, "Peanut allergy: dining with death," 2557, *New Scientist* (June 21, 2006).

36 N. Moran, "Ultimate allergy shot. Innovation: British company boasts of a vaccine with huge potential," *Independent* (Jan. 29, 1995).

37 D. Hamilton, "Silent treatment, how Genentech, Novartis stifled a promising drug, biotech firm tried to pursue peanut-allergy injection, but contract got in way," *The Wall Street Journal*, A1 (April 5, 2005).

38 Anon, "Center expands marketing of allergy product," *Health Industry Today* (July 1992).

39 In 1998, pharmaceutical giant Merck took a share in EpiPen sales through its ownership of Dey, L.P. EMI, an affiliate of Dey, L.P. became the exclusive distributor of EpiPen that was manufactured by Meridian Medical Technologies and marketed by King Pharmaceuticals a subsidiary of Meridian – Meridian was formed in 1996 by the merger of STI and Brunswick Biomedical. Dey assumed exclusive distribution rights in 2001. Majority of Dey Inc. was acquired in 1991 by Merck and then all of it by 1998. In 2008, 1.9 million Epipens were sold in the US, up more than 33% from 2003.

40 Anon, "Son's deadly allergy pits mom against school, *The Salt Lake Tribune* (April 4, 1994).

41 Anon, "Prestigious school rejects boy with peanut allergy," *Lexington Herald Leader* (April 15, 1995).

42 Anon, "Mom comes up with lifesaving badge," *Orange County Register* (May 5, 1994).

43 Wendy Harris, "Abnormal Response to Normal Things," *Professionally Speaking Magazine, Ontario College of Teachers* (Sept. 2000).

44 Anon, "Goodbye to the Goober," *Lifestyle, Newsweek* (Oct. 4, 1996).

45 Laura Lang, "Life threatening allergies spur peanut bans at Mass. Schools," *Education Week* (Nov. 6, 1996).

46 Anon, "Staple under fire: kids allergies bring schools' ban on peanut butter," *Arizona Daily Star* (Sept. 23, 1996).

47 S.M. Fletcher, "Snack peanuts purchase pattern," *Journal of Agricultural and Applied Economics* (April 1, 2002)

48 Emmanuel Foko*, Transforming Mature Industries into growth industries: the case of US peanuts* (Master of Agribusiness dissertation, Kansas State University, 2008).

49 Anon, "Group OKs GMO peanut research," *High Plains Journal* (Dec. 28, 2006). hpj.com

50 Anon, "NSW: peanut allergy case ends in multi-million dollar settlement," *AAP General News* (June 8, 2000).

51 The law is named for Sabrina Shannon, a 12-year-old girl who died in 2003 from anaphylactic shock after consuming cafeteria french fries contaminated by cheese.

52 Anon, "Mr. Peanut goes to court," *Journal of Law and Health* (March 22, 1999).

53 Anon, "Bullies use peanut butter to threaten kids with allergies," *Globe and Mail* (March 30, 2009).

54 Anon, "Man sentenced in peanut butter attack," *UPI* (Dec. 27, 2008).

55 Anon, "Warning of nut allergy 'hysteria'," *BBC News* online (Dec. 10 2008).

56 N. A. Christakis, "This allergy is just nuts," *British Medical Journal* (2008). This author is professor of Medical Sociology, Harvard Medical School.

57 Anon, "Call for specialist centres to tackle 'allergy epidemic'," *The Independent* (Sept. 26, 2007).

58 Anon, "The Food Allergy & Anaphylaxis Network (FAAN) and Verus Pharmaceuticals work together to raise awareness of food allergies," *PR Newswire* (Oct. 4, 2007). Verus produces the portable epinephrine dispensing Twinject, a competitor to Epipen.

59 C.A. Camargo, et al., "Regional differences in EpiPen prescriptions in the United States," *The Journal of Allergy and Clinical Immunology*, 120, 1 (July 2007): 131-136.

CHAPTER 2: Risk Factors

1 I. Dalal, et al., "Food allergy is a matter of geography after all: sesame as a major cause of severe IgE-mediated food allergic reactions among infants and young children in Israel," *European Journal of Allergy and Clinical Immunol.,* 57, 4 (March, 2002): 362-365.

2 S.H. Sicherer, et al. "Prevalence of peanut and tree nut allergy in the United States determined by means of a random digit dial telephone survey: a 5-year follow up study," *The Journal of Allergy and Clinical Immunology*, 112, 6, (Dec., 2003): 1203-1207

3 See Appendix.

4 S. Maleki, et al., "Is the low prevalence of peanut allergy in Israel due to hypoallergenic peanut products?" *J Allergy Clin Imunol.*, 115, 2 (Feb. 2005).

5 K. du Plessis, H. Steinman, "Practical aspects of adverse reactions to peanut," *Current Allergy & Clnical Immunology*, 17, 1 (March, 2004): 10-14.

6 Van Odijk, Op. cit.

7 Z. Kmietowicz, "Women warned to avoid peanuts during pregnancy and lactation," *BMJ*, 316 (June, 1998): 1926.

8 Ibid.

9 R. Hatahet, Op. cit.

10 P.W. Ewan, "Prevention of peanut allergy," *The Lancet*, 352, 9129 (Aug., 1998): 741-2.

11 G. Lack, et al., "Factors associated with the development of peanut allergy in childhood," *N Engl J Med.*, 348 (2003): 977-85.

12 T.C. Liang, *Maternal Dietary Modification for Prevention of Food Sensitisation* (Master of Nutrition and Dietetics dissertation, University of Wollongong, 2007).

13 T. Dean, "Government advice on peanut avoidance during pregnancy: is it followed correctly and what is the impact on sensitization?" *Journal Hum Nutr Diet*, 20 (2007): 95-99.

14 A. Muraro, et al. "Dietary prevention of allergic diseases in infants and small children part III," *Pediatr Allergy Immunol.*, 15 (2004): 291-307.

15 D. Moneret-Vautrin, et al., "Risk of milk formulas containing peanut oil contaminated with peanut allergens in infants with atopic dermatitis," *Pediatr Allergy Immunol.*, 5 (1994): 184-188.

16 G. De Montis, et al., "Sensitization to peanut and vitamin D oily preparations," *Lancet*, 341 (1993): 1411.

17 A. Cantani, "Anaphylaxis from peanut oil in infant feedings and medications*,*" *European Review of Medical and Pharmacological Sciences*, 2 (1998): 203-206.

18 G.K. Appelt, et al., "Breastfeeding and food avoidance are ineffective in preventing sensitization in high risk children," *The Journal of Allergy and Clinical Immunology*, 113, 2 (2004): 299.

19 *Memorandum by European Academy of Allergology and Clinical Immunology, The United Kingdom Parliament, House of Lord, Science and Technology, Minutes Evidence,* (2007).

20 G. Du Toit, et al., "Early consumption of peanuts in infancy is associated with a low prevalence of peanut allergy," *Journal of Allergy and Clinical Immunology*, 122 (Nov., 2008): 984-91.

2121 I. Dalal, et al. "The pattern of sesame sensitivity among infants and children," *Pediatr Allergy Immunol.*, 14, 4 (Aug., 2003): 312-6.

22 http://www.leapstudy.co.uk/study_about.html

23 G. Du Toit, "Learning Early about peanut allergy, The LEAP study," *The Newsletter of the British Society for Allergy & Clinical Immunology*, 8 (Autumn, 2006): 6.

24 J. Strid, et al., "A novel model of sensitization and oral tolerance to peanut protein," *Immunology*, 113, 3 (Nov., 2004): 293-303.

25 K. Bock, *Healing the New Childhood Epidemics, Autism, ADHD, Asthma, and Allergies* (New York, Random House, 2007)182.

26 "Allergy," *House of Lords, Science and Technology Committee, 6th Report of Session 2006-07*, I (Sept. 2007).

27 S. Sicherer, et al., "Food hypersensitivity and atopic dermatitis: pathophysiology, epidemiology, diagnosis and management," *J Allergy Clin Immunol.*,104, 3 (1999): S114-S122.

28 H. Sampson, "Managing peanut allergy," *BMJ*, 312 (1996): 1050-1

29 J. O'B Hourihane, et al. "Peanut allergy in relation to heredity, maternal diet, and other atopic diseases: results of a questionnaire survey, skin prick testing, and food challenges," *BMJ*, 313 (Aug., 1996): 518-521.

30 D.J. Hill, et al., "The frequency of food allergy in Australia and Asia," *Environmental Toxicology and Pharmacology*, 4, 1-2 (Nov. 1997): 101-110.

31 G. Du Toit, "Different prevalence of peanut allergy in children in Israel and UK is not due to differences in atopy," *Journal of Allergy and Clinical Immunology*, 117, 2, (Feb., 2006): Supplement.

32 T. Kemp T, et al., "Is infant immunization a risk factor for childhood asthma or allergy?" *Epidemiology*, 8 (1997): 678-680.

33 M. Odetn, et al., "Pertussis vaccination and asthma: is there a link?" *JAMA*, 272, 8 (Aug., 1994): 593. Quoted in A. Mercae, *From Immunology to social policy: epistemology and ethics in the creation and administration of paediatric vaccines* (Dissertation, University of Tasmania, April, 2003) http://eprints.utas.edu.au/31/1/Arlette_Mercae_Thesis.pdf; M. Odent, E. Culpin, "Effect of immunization status on asthma prevalence," *The Lancet*, 361, 9355 (Feb., 2003): 434.

34 H. Odelram, et al, "Immunoglobulin E and G responses to pertussis toxin after booster immunization in relation to atopy, local reactions and aluminium content of the vaccines," *Pediatric Allergy an Immunology*, 5, 2 (June, 2007): 118-123.

35 T. Shirakawa, et al., "The inverse association between tuberculin responses and atopic disorder," *Science*, 275, 5296 (Jan., 1997): 77-79.

36 J. Li, et al., "Absence of relationships between tuberculin responses and development of adult asthma with rhinitis and atopy," *Chest*, 133 (2008): 100-106.

37 R. Balicer, et al., Is childhood vaccination associated with asthma? A meta-analysis of observational studies," *Pediatrics*, 120, 5 (Nov. 2007): 1269-1277.

38 M. Profet, Op. cit., 26.

39 A. Mercae, Op. cit.

40 Cookson, et al., "Asthma, An epidemic in the absence of infection?" *Science Magazine*, 275, 5296 (Jan., 1997): 41-442.

41 M. Wjst, "The Triple T Allergy Hypothesis," *Clinical & Developmental Immunology*, 11, 2 (June, 2004): 175-180.

42 M. Ryan, et al., "Distinct T-cell subtypes induced with whole cell and acellular pertussis vaccines in children," *Immunology*, 93 (1998): 1-10. Quoted in A. Mercae, Op. cit., 24.

43 D. Granoff, "Are serological responses to acellular pertussis antigens sufficient criteria to ensure that new combination vaccines are effective for prevention of disease?" *Developments in Biological*

Standardisation, 89 (1997): 379-89. Quoted in A. Mercae, Op. cit., 24.

44 J.M. van Oosterhout, A.C. Motta, "Th1/Th2 paradigm: not seeing the forest for the trees?" *Eur Respir J.,* 25 (2005): 591-593.

45 T.D. Green, et al. "Clinical Characteristics of Peanut-Allergic Children: Recent Changes," *Pediatrics,* 120, 6 (Dec. 2007): 1304-1310.

46 Ibid.

47 Green, Op. cit., 8.

48 Ibid.

49 S. Sicherer, et al. "Clinical features of acute allergic reactions to peanut and tree nuts in children," *Pediatrics,* 102, 1 (1997).

50 T. Vander Leek, et al., "The natural history of peanut allergy in young children and its association with serum peanut-specific IgE," *J Pediatr.,* 137 (2000): 749-755; H. Skolnik, et al., "The natural history of peanut allergy," *J Allergy Clin Immunol.,* 107 (2007): 367-374.

51 Mullins, Op. cit., 4.

52 S. Sicherer, et al. "Prevalence of peanut and tree nut allergy in the United States determined by means of a random digit dial telephone survey: a 5 year follow up study." *Journal of Allergy and Clin Immunol.,* 112 (2003): 1203-1207.

53 M. D. Kogan, et al., "Prevalence of parent-reported diagnosis of autism spectrum disorder among children in the US, 2007," *Pediatrics* (Oct. 5, 2009).

54 Sex ratio, the proportion of male to female births, is indicative of reproductive health in all animals. A dramatic decline in male births in the Aamjiwnaang First Nation community between 1999 and 2003 startled researchers. Ratio of births in this period was about 33% boys and 67% girls, a ratio of 2:1. This community of 850 people resides on the St. Clair River near Sarnia, Ontario. It is believed that the trend is the result of exposures to endocrine-disrupting effluent and emissions of nearby petrochemical plants. The toxins include phthalates, a plasticizer to which humans are exposed daily in soft plastics, skin creams, shampoo, hair condition and more.

55 R. Lockey, "Mechanisms of Anaphylaxis," *Life-Threatening Allergy, an Homage to Von Pirquet,* Mp3 lecture, World Allergy Forum, Vienna (June 11, 2006).

56 P.J. Hannaway, et al., "Differences in race ethnicity, and socioeconomic status in school children dispensed injectable epinephrine in 3 Massachusetts school districts," *Ann Allergy Asthma Immunol.,* 95, 2 (Aug., 2005): 143-8.

57 C. Kuehni, et al., "Food intolerance and wheezing in young South Asian and white children: Prevalence and clinical significance," *The Journal of Allergy and Clinical Immunology,* 118 (2006): 528-30.

58 F. Cataldo, et al., "Are food intolerances and allergies increasing in immigrant children coming from developing countries?" *Pediatric Allergy and Immunology,* 17 (2006): 364-69.

59 C. Kuehni, Op. cit.

60 M. Eggesbo, et al., "Is Delivery by Cesarean section a risk factor for food allergy?" *Journal of Allergy and Clinical Immunology,* 112, 2 (2003): 420-426.

61 B. Laubereau, et al., "Caesarean section and gastrointestinal symptoms, atopic dermatitis and sensitization during the first year of life," *Archives of Disease in Childhood,* 89, 11 (Nov., 2004): 993-997.

62 M. Eggesbo, "Cesarean delivery and cowmilk allergy/intolerance," *Allergy,* 60, 9 (Aug., 2005): 1172-73.

63 M. Kuitunen, et al., "Probiotics prevent IgE associated allergy until age 5 years in cesarean-delivered children but not in the total cohort," *Journal of Allergy and Clinical Immunology,* 10 (2008): 1016.

64 M.L. Moore, "Reducing the rate of Cesarean birth," *J Perinat Educ.,* 11, 2 (Spring, 2002): 41-43.

65 J.A. Martin, "Births: Final data for 2006," *National Vital Statistics Reports,* CDC, 57, 7

66 A. Steinberg, *Encyclopedia of Jewish Medical Ethics* (Israel, Feldheim Publishers, 2003) 170.

67 R. Gonen, "Obstetricians' Opinions regarding patient choice in cesarean delivery," *Obstetrics & Gynecology,* 99, 4 (April, 2002): 577-580.

68 C. Weissman, et al., "The Israeli anesthesiology physician workforce," *IMAJ,* 8 (April 2006).

69 I. Dalal, et al., "Food allergy is a matter of geography after all: sesame as a major cause of severe IgE mediated food allergic reactions among infants and young children in Israel," *Allergy,* 57, 4 (April, 2002): 362-5.

70 D. Aaronov, et al, "Natural history of food allergy in infants and children in Israel," *Ann Allergy Asthma Immunol.,* 101, 6 (Dec., 2008): 637-40.

71 J. O'B Hourihane, "The prevalence of peanut allergy in British children at school entry age in 2003," *Foodbase, Food Standards Agency* (31/05/2006).

72 A. F. Dioun, et al. "Is maternal age at delivery related to childhood food allergy? *Pediatr Allergy Immunol.*,14, 4 (Aug., 2003): 307-311.

73 http://www.allcountries.org/uscensus/90_cesarean_section_deliveries_by_age_of.html

74 Highlights from EAACI 2009, XXVIII Congress of he European Academy of Allergy and Clinical Immunology, June 6-10, Warsaw, Poland.

http://www.theucbinstituteofallergy.com/Images/EAACI_2009.pdf Also, E. von Mutius, et al., "Prevalence of asthma and atopy in two areas of West and East Germany," *Am J Respir Crit Care Med.*,149 (1994): 358-364.

75 D. Strachan, "Socioeconomic factors and the development of allergy," *Toxicol Lett.*, 86 (1996): 199-203.

76 C. Roehr, et al., "Food allergy and non-allergic food hypersensitivity in children and adolescents," *Clin Exp Allergy*, 34, 1 (Oct., 2004): 1534-41.

77 A. Mehl, et al., "Anaphylactic reactions in children – a questionnaire-based survey in Germany," *Allergy*, 60, 11 (2005): 1440-1445.

78 A. Sheikh, et al. "Anaphylaxis discharge rates by regional health authority, per 100,000 discharges," *Clin Exp Allergy*, 31 (2001): 15671-76.

79 G. Lack, et al., "Factors associated with the development of peanut allergy in childhood," *The New England Journal of Medicine*, 348 (March, 2003): 977-985.

80 M.P. Oryszczyn, et al., "Head circumference at birth and maternal factors related to cord blood total IgE," *Clin Exp Allergy*, 29, 3 (March, 1999): 334-41.

81 V. Emerton (ed.), *Food allergy and intolerance: current issues and concerns*, (Great Britain, Royal Society of Chemistry, 2002) 11.

82 J. O'B Hourihane, et al., "Peanut allergy in relation to heredity, maternal diet, and other atopic diseases: results of a questionnaire survey, skin prick testing, and food challenges," *BMJ*, 313 (1996): 518-521.

83 Ibid.

84 G. Lack, et al., "Factors associated with the development of peanut allergy in childhood," *The New England Journal of Medicine*, 348 (March 13, 2003): 977-985.

85 J. O'B. Hourihane, Op. cit.

86 S. Sicherer, et al., "Genetics of peanut allergy: a twin study," *Journal of Allergy and Clinical Immunology*, 106, 1 (July 2000): 53-56.

87 B. Bjorksten, "Genetic and Environmental Risk Factors for the Development of Food Allergy," *Curr Opin Allergy Clin Immunol.*, 5, 3 (2005): 249-253.

88 Xiu-min Li, et al., "Strain-dependent induction of allergic sensitization caused by peanut allergen DNA immunization in Mice," *The Journal of Immunology*, 162 (1999): 3045-3052.

89 K. Bock, Op. cit.

90 Ibid, 177.

91 Ibid, 51.

92 M. Hitti, "Childhood vaccination rates high," *Web MD Health News* (Sept. 4, 2008). http://children.webmd.com/vaccines/news/20080904/childhood-vaccination-rates-high

93 Letter from Marlyn B. Maloney and Christopher H. Smith, Members of Congress in a letter to Hon. Kathleen Sebelius, Secretary, Health and Human Services, June 10, 2009.

94 Devi Lockwood, "Is there a link between vaccinations and peanut allergies," *Connecticut Science Fair* (2007) http://www.avoidingmilkprotein.com/vacandpea.htm

95 Bock, Op. cit., 57. Both Bock and Lockwood point out this CDC rationalization.

96 H. Skolnick, et al., "The natural history of peanut allergy," *J Allergy Cli Immunol.*, 107 (2001): 367-374.

97 Ibid.

98 J. O'B. Hourihane, et al., "Resolution of peanut allergy: case-control study," *BMJ*, 316 (1998): 1271-1275.

99 G. Du Toit, et al., "Early consumption of peanuts in infancy is associated with a low prevalence of peanut allergy," *Journal of Allergy and Clinical Immunology*, 122 (Nov., 2008): 984-91.

100 G. Du Toit, "Learning Early about peanut allergy, The LEAP study," *The Newsletter of the British Society for Allergy & Clinical Immunology*, 8 (Autumn, 2006): 6.
101 J. O'B Hourihane, et al., "Resolution of peanut allergy following bone marrow transplantation for primary immunodeficiency," *Allergy*, 60, 4 (April, 2005): 536 537.

CHAPTER 3: Theories

1 L. Hammarstrom, C. Smith, "Immunologlobulin subclass distribution of specific antibodies in allergic patients," *Allergy*, 42 (1987): 529-534.
2 http://www.nationaljewish.org/healthinfo/conditions/allergy/index.aspx National Jewish Health (August, 2009).
3 J. Woodfolk, "Selective roles and dysregulation of interleukin-10 in allergic disease," *Current Allergy & Asthma Reports*, 6, 1 (Jan. 2006): 40-46.
4 Reneé Dubos, *The Dreams of Reason: Science and Utopias* (New York, 1961) 71.
5 Lack, G. et al "Factors Associated with the Development of Peanut Allergy in Childhood," *The New England Journal of Medicine*, 11, 348 (March 13, 2003): 977-985.
6 R. Weeks, "Peanut oil in medications," *The Lancet*, 348, 9029: 759-760. The World Standard Drug Database listed skin creams that contain peanut oil including: Calamine oily lotion; Eczederm cream; Hydromol cream; Hewletts cream, Kamillosan ointment; Masse cream; Siopel cream; Zinc cream; Polytar emollient; and more
7 Lack, Op. cit.
8 J. Strid, J. O'B Hourihane, et al., "Epicutaneous exposure to peanut protein prevents oral tolerance and enhances allergic sensitization," *Clin Exp.*, (June, 2005).
9 Peeters et al, "Peanut allergy: Sensitization by peanut oil-containing local therapeutics seems unlikely," *J Allergy Clin Immunol* (May 2004).
10 Smith, Op. cit., 97.
11 U.S. FDA "Listing of Food Additive Status", (March 2009). See also http://www.cosmeticsdatabase.com/ingredient.php?ingred06=700482&nothanks=1
12 A. Olszewski, et al., "Isolation and characterization of proteic allergens in refined peanut oil," *Clin Exp Allergy*, 28, 7 (July, 1998): 850-9. "In conclusion, we have demonstrated the presence of allergenic proteins in crude and refined peanut oil. These proteins are the same size as two allergens previously described in peanut protein extracts."
13 G. Lack, et al., "Avon Longitudinal Study of Parents and Children Study Team. Factors associated with the development of peanut allergy in childhood," *N Engl J Med*, 348 (2003): 977-85.
14 http://www.cfsan.fda.gov/~Dms/Alrgn.Html
15 http://www.whc-oils.com/refined-peanut-oil.html
16 The USP-NF is a book of public pharmacopeial standards containing standards for medicines, excipients, etc. In it is a "procedure" for refining peanut oil http://www.usp.org/pdf/EN/monoRedesign/NF-Monos-I-Z.pdf
17 J.B. Greig & Joint FAO/WHO Expert Committee on Food Additives, "Potential allergenicity of refined food products, peanut oils and soya bean oils*," WHO Food Additive Series, International Program on Chemical Safety*, 44 (2000): 8. http://www.inchem.org/documents/jecfa/jecmono/v44jec11.htm
18 Ibid.
19 G. De Montis, et al., "Sensitization to peanut and vitamin D oily preparations," Lancet 341 (1993): 1411.
20 D.A. Moneret-VAutrin, et al., "Risk of milk formulas containing peanut oil contaminated with peanut allergens in infants with atopic dermatitis," *Pediatr Allergy Immunol.*, 5, 3 (Dec., 1993): 184-188.
21 A. Cantani, "Anaphylaxis from peanut oil in infant feedings and medications," *European Review of Medical and Pharmacological Sciences*, 2 (1998): 203-206.
22 D.A. Moneret-Vautrin, et al., Op. cit.
23 "Refined Peanut Oil NF, FDA Registered, CGMP Proven Quality, All Natural," Welch, Holm & Clark Col, Inc. http://www.whc-oils.com/refined-peanut-oil.html
24 S. Sicherer S., H. Sampson, "Peanut allergy: Emerging concepts and approaches for a apparent epidemic," *Journal of Allergy and Clinical Immunology*, 120, 3 (Sept., 2007): 491-503.

25 S.H. Sicherer, et al., "Prevalence of peanut and tree nut allergy in the United States determined by means of a random digit dial telephone survey: a 5-year follow up study," *JACI*, 112, 6 (Dec. 2003): 1203-1207.

26 J. Bernhisel-Broadbent, H. Sampson, "Cross-allergenicity in the legume botanical family in children with food hypersensitivity," *J Allergy Clin Immunol.*, 83 (1989): 435-40.

27 R.J. Dearman, I. Kimber, "Proteins as allergens: a toxicological perspective," *Food allergy and intolerance: current issues and concerns* (Great Britain, Royal Society of Chemistry, 2002)14 ff.

28 M. Frieri, B. Kettelhut (ed.), *Food Hypersensitivity and adverse reactions: a practical guide for diagnosis Clinical Allergy and Immunology* (CRC Press, 1999) 84.

29 S. D. Kelleher, et al. "Functional Chicken Muscle Protein Isolates…" *53rd Annual Reciprocal Meat Conference, American Meat Science Association* (2000) www.meatscience.org Beef serum albumin and muscle protein (BSA and BGG) has a molecular weight of between 17 and 66 kD; albumin in egg 45 kD.

30 S.J. Maleki, et al., "Structure of the Major Peanut Allergen Ara h 1 May Protect IgE-Binding Epitopes from Degradation," *J Immunol.*, 164, 11 (June, 2000): 5844-9.

31 D.J. DeNoon, "CDC: 4% of US Children New Suffer Food Allergies," MedicineNet.com (Oct. 22, 2008)

32 K. Beyer, et al., "Effects of cooking methods on peanut allergenicity," *J Allergy Clin Immuno.l*, 107 (2001): 1077-81.

33 M. Khodoun, et al., "Peanuts can contribute to anaphylactic shock by activating complement," *J Allergy Clin Immunol.*, 123, 2 (Feb., 2009): 333-351.

34 S.J. Koppelman, "Quantification of major peanut allergens Ara h 1 and Ara h 2 in the peanut varieties Runner, Spanish, Virginia, and Valencia, bred in different parts of the world," *Allergy*, 56, 2 (Feb., 2001): 132-7.

35 G. Du Toit, et al., "Early consumption of peanuts in infancy is associated with a low prevalence of peanut allergy," *Journal of Allergy and Clinical Immunology* (November, 2008).

36 Charles Richet, *The Nobel Prize in Physiology or Medicine 1913, Nobel Lecture* (Dec. 11, 1913). http://nobelprize.org/nobel_prizes/medicine/laureates/1913/richet-lecture.html

37 M. Profet, "The Function of Allergy: Immunological Defense Against Toxins," *The Quarterly Review of Biology*, 66, 1 (1991).

38 Profet, Op. cit., 38.

39 R. Fischer, et al., "Oral and Nasal Sensitization Promote distinct immune responses and reactivity in a mouse model of peanut allergy," *American Journal of Pathology*, 167 (2005): 1621-1630; F. van Wijk, et al., "The CD28/CTLA-4-B7 signaling pathway is involved in both allergic sensitization ad tolerance induction to orally administered peanut proteins," *The Journal of Immunology*, 178 (2007): 6894-6900.

40 J. W. Coleman, M. Blanca, "Mechanisms of drug allergy", *Immunology Today*, 19, 5 (May 1998): 196-198; A. Cantani, *Pediatric allergy, asthma and immunology*, (Germany, Springer, 2008) 1150; A.L. Schocket (ed.), *Clinical management of uticaria and anaphylaxis*, (US, Marcel Dekker, Inc., 1993) 120.

41 M. Frieri, B. Kettelhut, *Food hypersensitivity and adverse reactions: a practical guide for diagnosis* (CRC Press, 1999) 81.

42 A. Cantani, Op. cit., 214.

43 Profet, Op. cit., 35.

44 Ibid, 36.

45 O.L. Frick, D.L. Brooks, "Immunologloglobulin E antibodies to pollens augmented in dogs by virus vaccines," *Am. J. Vet. Res.*, 44 (1983):440-445. Quoted in Profet, Op. cit., 46.

46 S. Scrivener, et al. "Independent effects of intestinal parasite infection and domestic allergen exposure on risk of wheeze in Ethiopia: a case-control study," *Lancet*, 358 (2001): 1493-1499.

47 A.H. Van den Biggelaar, et al., "The prevalence of parasite infestation and house dust mite sensitization in Gabonese schoolchildren," *Int Arch Allergy Immunol.*,126 (2001): 231-238.

48 D.E. Elliot, et al., "Helminths as governors of immune-mediated inflammation," *International Journal for Parasitology* (2007).

49 R. M. Maizels, M. Yazdanbakhsh, "Immune regulation by helminth parasites: cellular and molecularl mechanisms," *Nature Reviews, Immunology*, 3 (Sept. 2003): 733.

50 E.A. Sabin et al. "Impairment of tetanus thoxoid-sepcific Th1-like immune responses in humans infected with Schistosoma mansoni," *J Infect. Dis.*, 173 (1996): 269-272; A.J. Macdonald, et al. "A

novel, helminth-derived immuostimulant enhances human recall response to hepatitis C virus and tetanus toxoid and is dependent on CD56+ cells for its action," *Clin Exp Immunol.*,152 (2008): 265-273.

51 Klaus Erb, "Can helminths or helminth-derived products be used in humans to prevent or treat allergic diseases?" *Trends in Immunology*, 30, 2 (Feb. 2009): 75-82.

52 M. Yazdanbakhsh, S. Wahyuni, "The role of helminth infections in protection from atopic disorders," *Current Opinion in Allergy and Clinical Immunology*, 5 (2005): 386-391.

53 Ibid.

54 K.J. Erb,"Helminths, allergic disorders and IgE-mediated immune responses: where do we stand?" *European Journal of Immunology*, 37, 5 (April, 2007): 1170-1173

55 Ibid.

56 Profet, Op. cit., 48.

57 B. Ogilivie, V. Jones. "Immunity in the parasitic relationships between helminths and hosts," *Prog. Allergy*, 17 (1973): 93-144.

58 M.L. Baeza, et al. "Anisakis simplex allergy: a murine model of anaphylaxis induced by parasitic proteins displays a mixed Th1Thx pattern," *British Society for Immunology*, 142, 3 (Dec.2005): 433-440.

59 D.A. Johnson, "Is H. Pylori infection protective against asthma and allergies?" *Gastroenterology*, 57 (May, 2008): 561; Y. Chen, M.J. Blaser, "Inverse associations of Helicobacter pylori with asthma and allergy," *Arch Intern Med*, 167 (2007): 821-827

60 P.G. Engelkirk, *Laboratory diagnosis of infectious diseases* (Philadelphia, Wolters Kluwer Health, 2008) 596.

61 B.E. Zacharia, P. Sherman, "Allergies, helminths, and cancer," *Med Hypotheses*, 60 (Sept., 2005): 1-5.

62 A. Gosline, "Peanut allergy: dining with death," *New Scientist*, 2557 (June 21, 2006). http://www.newscientist.com/article/mg19025571.500-peanut-allergy-dining-with-death.html?page=3

63 L. Chiu, et al. "Estimation of the sensitization rate to peanut by prick skin test in the general population: results from the National Health and Nutrition Examination Survey, 1980-1994," *J Allergy Clin Immunol.*,107 (2001): S192.

64 Anon, "Current Trends in Allergic Reactions: a multidisciplinary approach t patient management," *Clinician, National Institute of Allergy and Infectious diseases of the National Institutes of Health, US Dept. of Health and Human Services*, 21, 3 (Sept. 2003).

65 D.P. Strachan, "Family size, infection and atopy: the first decade of the hygiene hypothesis," *Thorax*, 55 (2000): S2-S10.

66 Ibid, S8.

67 M. Akdis, et al. "T regulatory cells in allergy: novel concepts in the pathogenesis, prevention and treatment of allergic diseases," *J Allergy Clin Immuol.* 116, 5 (Nov., 2005): 961-8.

68 Profet, Op. cit., 46.

69 O.L. Frick, D.L. Brooks, "Immunolglobulin E antibodies to pollens augmented in dogs by virus vaccines," *Am. J. Vet. Res.*, 44 (1983):440-445. Quoted in Profet, Op. cit., 46.

70 M. Yazdanbakhsh, Op. cit.

71 J. Diamond, "The Worst Mistake in the History of the Human Race", *Discover Magazine* (May, 1987). See also J. Diamond, *Guns, Germs and Steel* (2005).

PART 2: A History of Mass Allergy

CHAPTER 4: Re-discovering anaphylaxis

1 J. Ring, H. Behrendt, "Anaphylaxis and Anaphylactoid Reactions," *Clinical Reviews in Allergy and Immunology*, 7, 4 (Dec., 1999).

2 L. H. Freude, J. Rejaunier, *The Complete Idiot's Guide to Food Allergies* (New York: Penguin Group, 2003)14.

3 Mark Jackson, *Allergy, The History of a Modern Malady* (London: Reaktion Books, 2007) 28.

4 Jared Diamond, "The Worst Mistake in the History of the Human Race", *Discover Magazine* (May, 1987).

5 Ibid.

6 Richard Preston, *The Demon in the Freezer, a true story* (New York: Random House, 2002) 24.

7 S. Riedel, "Edward Jenner and the history of smallpox and vaccination," *Proceedings (Bayl Univ Med Cent)*, 18, 1 (Jan., 2005): 21-25.

8 Edward Jenner, *An inquiry into the causes and effects of the variolae vaccinae* (London, 1798).

9 J.G. Rigau-Perez, "The Introduction of Smallpox Vaccine in 1803 and the Adoption of Immunization as a Government Function in Puerto Rico," *Hispanic American Historical Review*, 69, 3 (1989): 393–423, quoted in A. Minna Stern, H. Markel, "The History of Vaccines and Immunization: Familiar Patterns, New Challenges," *Health Affairs*, 24, 3 (2005): 611-621.

10 H. Davies, "Ethical reflections on Edward Jenner's experimental treatment," *Journal of Medical Ethics*, 33 (2007): 174-176. The inoculation technique was developed in China, Africa and India well before the 18th century when English aristocrat Lady Mary Wortley Montague introduced it to Europe. Lady Mary's brother had died of smallpox and she herself had suffered an episode that disfigured her face. Convinced that inoculation was the lesser of two evils, she had both her children treated. Subsequent inoculations of prisoners and orphans were deemed a success when no one died. Ultimately in 1722, the two daughters of the Princess of Wales were inoculated without incident. With this star endorsement, the technique began to gain acceptance.

11 D. Baxby, "Smallpox vaccination techniques; from knives and forks to needles and pins," *Vaccine*, 20, 16 (May, 2002): 2140-2149.

12 D.A. Henderson, "Edward Jenner's vaccine," *Public Health Reports* (Mar/April 1997): 112.

13 J. B. Tucker, *Scourge: The Once and Future Threat of Smallpox* (New York: Atlantic Monthly Press, 2001).

14 T. Reimer, *Smallpox and Vaccination in the Civil War: National Museum of Civil War Medicine* (NMCWM Press, 2004). http:www.civilwarmed.org

15 I. Berry, R. Martin, *The Pharmaceutical Regulatory Process* (Informa Health Care, 2008) 6.

16 R. Porter, *Disease, Medicine and Society in England, 1550-1860* (Cambridge U. Press, 1995) 42.

17 P.W. Laird, *Advertising progress: American business and the rise of consumer marketing* (Baltimore: Johns Hopkins University Press 1998) 480. Quoted in Kalman Applbaum "Pharmaceutical Marketing and the Invention of the Medical Consumer," *PLoS Med (Public Library of Science)* 3, 4 (April, 2006).

18 David Lilienfeld, "The First Pharmacoepidemiologic Investigations national drug safety policy in the United States, 1901-1902," *Perspectives in Biology and Medicine*, 51, 2 (Spring 2008). Renown psychiatrist Sigmund Freud quoted articles from this publication and made financial arrangements with Parke, Davis and Merck to support research in *On Coca* 1884. In this publication he supported the beneficial effects of cocaine for many problems including morphine addiction.

19 Ibid.

20 L. Glambos, J. Eliot Sewell, *Networks of Innovation: Vaccine Development at Merck, Sharp and Dohme, and Mulford, 1895-1995* (New York: Cambridge U. Press, 1995). When Mulford went into decline in the 1920s it was purchased in 1929 by Sharp & Dohme. This company merged with Merck in 1953. Merck dominated the marketplace in 2009.

21 Anne Hardy, *The Epidemic Streets: infectious disease and the rise of preventive medicine, 1856-1900* (Oxford U. Press, 1993) 83.

22 William Bynum, *Science and the Practice of Medicine in the Nineteenth Century* (Cambridge University Press, 1994) 164.

23 Ibid,161.

24 Anon, "Horse 397, Condemned as useless, proved worth $175,000," *The New York Times* (June 7, 1914).

25 F.J. Grunbacher. "Behring's discovery of Dip and tetanus anti-toxins", *Immunology Today*, 13 (1992):188-90. Quoted in Jackson, Op. cit., 31.

26 R.A. Kondratas, "Biologics Control Act of 1902," *The Early Years of Federal Food and Drug Control* (1982) 8-27. Quoted in Lilienfeld, Op. cit.

27 I. Berry, R. Martin, *The Pharmaceutical Regulatory Process* (Informa Health Care, 2008) 3.

28 Ibid, 5.

29 Anon, "Attorney General Acts Against Drug Trust, Seeks an Injunction to Prevent Control of Prices, Suit Brought in Indiana, Proprietary and Wholesale and Retail Druggists' Associations Named as Defendants, Conspiracy Charged," *The New York Times* (May 10, 1906).

30 Stuart Anderson, *Making Medicines: a brief history of pharmacy and pharmaceuticals* (Pharmaceutical Press, 2005) 156.

31 Intravenous injection and infusion began as early as 1670.

32 Gary Matsumoto, *Vaccine A* (Basic Books, 2004) 26.

33 K. Stratton, et al., *Adverse Events Associated with Childhood Vaccines* (National Academies Press, 1994) 223-224.

34 E.A. Belongia, A.L. Naleway, "Smallpox Vaccine: The Good, the Bad and the Ugly," *Clin Med Res*,1, 2 (April, 2003):87-92. The authors of this article attempt to show that the "vaccine is a critical tool for controlling smallpox ("the good"), despite a relatively higher risk of complications in some individuals ("the bad"). The "ugly" refers not to the vaccine, but to the potential reintroduction of smallpox more than 20 years after its eradication."

35 M. Hassani, et al., "Vaccines for the prevention of diseases caused by potential bioweapons," *Clinical Immunology*, 111, 1 (April 2004): 1-15.

36 Vaughan, 46.

37 A. Nelson, C. Horsburgh, *Pathology of Emerging Infections 2* (ASM Press, 1998) 146.

38 "M. Meddow Bayly, "Some Little-Understood Effects of Serum Therapy," *Medical World* (April 6, 1934).

39 Clemens von Pirquet, "On the Theory of Infectious Diseases," (April,1903). Cited by Jackson, Op. cit., 35-36.

40 C. Von Pirquet, B. Schick, *Serum Sickness*, (1905). Translated by B. Schick (Baltimore, 1951).

41 C. von Pirquet, "Allergie", *Munchener Medizinische Wochenschrift* (1906). Cited in Jackson, Op. cit., 37.

42 Vaughan, Op. cit., 46.

43 Nadja Durbach, *Bodily Matters: The Anti-vaccination Movement in England, 1853-1907* (Durham: Duke University Press, 2005) 97.

44 Ibid,100.

45 G.T. Keusch, "The History of nutrition: malnutrition, infection and immunity," *J Nutr.*, 133, 1 (Jan., 2003): 336S-340S. It less well publicized that western nutrition science grew concurrent with biomedical research. Knowledge of host nutritional status and immunity was well established. Food as a cure or prevention for disease was a concept explored by Hippocrates in 400 BC who encouraged his students to "let thy food be thy medicine". The term "vitamins" was coined by Dr. Casmir Funk in 1912. In 1930, William Rose discovered essential amino acids, building blocks of proteins. The cyclical relationship between poor nutrition or malnutrition such as the severe "kwashiorkor" resulting from insufficient dietary protein and the spread of infectious disease was not well documented before 1959.

46 Eleanora McBean, *The Poisoned Needle* (Health Research Books, 1957, 1993) 10. Online http://www.scribd.com/doc/12983463/The-Poisoned-Needle-by-Eleanor-Mcbean

47 George Bernard Shaw, "Preface", *Doctor's Dilemma* (1909).

48 Richet, Op. cit.

49 Ibid.

50 Ibid.

51 Richet noticed that anaphylactized animals even when they seem in perfect health have leucocytes that often exceed 200.

52 A. Besredka, P Roux, *Anaphylaxis and Anti-Anaphylaxis* (London, Heinemann, 1919) 18.

53 Richet, Op. cit.

54 Ibid.

55 Vaughan, Op. cit., 110.

56 Ilana Lowy "On guinea pigs, dogs an dmen: anaphylaxis and the study of biological individuality, 1902-1939," *Studies in History and Philosophy of Science Part C*, 34, 3 (Sept. 2003): 399-423.

57 A. Schofield, "A Case of Egg Poisoning," *Lancet* (1908): 716.

58 O. Schloss, "A Case of Allergy to Common Foods," *Am J Dis Child*, 3 (1912): 341.

59 J. Hettwer, R. Kriz, "Absorption of Undigested Protein from the Alimentary Tract as Determined by the Direct Anaphylaxis Test," *American Journal of Physiology*, 73 (1925): 539-546.

60 Clinical allergy focused on environment allergies and de-sensitization through injection. British allergists John Freeman and Leonard Noon published accounts of injecting increasing doses of an extract of pollen to reduce sensitivity to same in 1911. Others experimented with desensitization: B.

Keston, et al., "Oral Desensitization to Common Foods," *J Allergy*, 6 (1935): 431; T.G. Randolph, "Allergy as a Causative Factor of Fatigue, Irritability, and Behavioral Problems of Children," *J Pediatrics* , 31(1947): 560-572.

61 W.T. Longcope, F.M. Rachemann, "Severe renal insufficiency associated with attacks of urticaria in hypersensitive individuals," *Journal of Urology*, 1(1917): 351; W. Duke, "Food allergy as a cause of abdominal pain," *Arch Int Med*, 28 (1921):151; W. Duke, "Food allergy as a cause of bladder pain," *Ann Clin Med.*, 1,(1922): 117; W.Duke, "Meniere's syndrome caused by allergies," *JAMA*, 81 (1923): 2179.

62 Vaughan, Op. cit., 109.

63 S. Plotkin, et al, *Vaccines* (Elsevier Health Sciences, 2008) 6.

64 Vaughan, Op. cit., 46.

65 A. Besredka, *Anaphylaxis and Anti-Anaphylaxis and Their Experimental Foundations* (London: William Henkmann (Medical Books) Ltd., 1919).

66 H.M. Gezon, et al., "A new repository penicillin (a form of aqueous penicillin G procaine) in infants and children," *Pediatrics*, 4 (July, 1949): 15; A. B. Cannon, et al., "Maintenance of penicillin blood levels after a single intramuscular injection of penicillin in various oils," *Science*, 104, 2705 (Nov. 1946): 414-415.

67 W.G. Myers, "The urinary excretion of penicillin after ingestion with and without adjuvants and following intramuscular injection," *The Ohio Journal of Science*, XLVI, 2 (March, 1946): 53-64. https://kb.osu.edu/dspace/bitstream/1811/3508/1/V46N02_053.pdf

68 Judy Hankins, *Infusion Therapy in Clinical Practice* (Elsivier, 2001) 3.

69 Francoise Nielloud, Gilberte Marti-Mestres, *Pharmaceutical emulsions and suspensions* (CRC Press, 2000) 236.

70 E.J. Coulson, J.R. Spies, "The Immunochemistry of allergens III, Anaphylactogenic potency of the electrophoretic fractionation products of CS-1A from Cottonseed," *The Journal of Immunology*, 46 (1943): 367-376.

71 Vaughan, Op. cit., 155.

72 Earlier articles in literature cited in F.M. Atkins, et al., "Cottonseed hypersensitivity: new concerns over an old problem," *J Allergy Clin Immunol.*, 82, 2 (Aug. 1988): 242-50.

73 T.G. Randolph, "Cottonseed protein vs. cottonseed oil sensitivity; a case of cottonseed oil sensitivity," *Ann Allergy*, 8,1 (Jan-Feb., 1950): 5-10.

74 National Cottonseed Products Association and the US Federal Security Agency, *Allergy to cottonseed and other oilseeds and their edible derivatives. Excerpts from testimony before the Administrator, Federal Security Agency in the matter of fixing and establishing definitions and standards of identity for mayonnaise, French dressing, and related salad dressings (Docket FDC-51) Public hearings held at Washington, D.C., Nov. 18-1947 and January 6 to 8, 1948,* (Memphis, National Cottonseed Products Assn., 1948).

75 Anon, "Allergy to cottonseed and other oil seeds and the edible derivatives," *Calif Med.*, 71, 5 (Nov., 1949): 384.

76 Garry Nall, "Encyclopedia of Oklahoma history & culture," *Oklahoma Historical Society* (undated). http://digital.library.okstate.edu/encyclopedia/entries/C/CO066.html

77 Lynette Boney Wrenn, *Cinderella of the New South: A History of the Cottonseed Industry, 1855-1955* (Knoxville, University of Tennessee Press, 1995).

78 Based on on-line review of medical journals as well as information in F.M. Atkins, et al., "Cottonseed hypersensitivity: new concerns over an old problem," *J Allergy Clin Immunol.*, 82, 2 (Aug. 1988): 242-50.

79 F.W. Denny, et al., "Comparative effects of penicillin, auremycin and terramycin on streptococcal tonsillitis and pharyngitis," *Pediatrics*, 11 (Jan., 1953): 7-14.

CHAPTER 5: The History of Peanut Allergy

1 The story of Patricia Malone, published in the NY Journal American won a Pulitzer Prize in 1944.

2 David Wilson, *In Search of Penicillin* (Knopf, 1976).

3 David Greenwood, *Antimicrobial Drugs, Chronicle of a Twentieth Century Medical Triumph* (Oxford University Press, 2008) 120. Through the 1940s, efforts to produce the same wonder drug in

Germany, Ausria, Czechoslovakia and other countries had yielded results but were delayed with the end of WW II.

4 Monroe J. Romansky, George E. Rittman, "A method of prolonging the action of penicillin," *Science*, 100, 2592 (Sept. 1, 1944): 196-198.

5 T. Guthe, et al., "Untoward penicillin reactions," *Bulletin, World Health Organization*, 19, 3 (1958): 427-501.

6 P.C. Trussell et al., "Duration of Effective Blood levels following administration of penicillin in peanut oil and beeswax," *Canad. M.A.J.*, 57 (Oct. 1947): 387; R.V. Platou, et al., "Round Table Discussion on Antibiotics," *Pediatrics*, 1 (Feb., 1948): 270-287; B.M. Kagan, et al., "Studies of Penicillin in Pediatrics: III, Procaine Penicillin G in Sesame Oil, in Peanut Oil with 2% Aluminum Monostearate and in Water with Sodium Carboxmethylcellulose," *Pediatrics*, 5, 4 (April 1950): 664-671.

7 G. Hildick-Smith, et al., "Penicillin Regimens in Pediatric Practice: Study of Blood Levels," *Pediatrics* (Jan. 1950): 97-113.

8 T.E. Roy, Antibiotics and iatrogenic disease," *Pediatrics*, 22 (1958); 167.

9 Guthe, Op. cit.

10 Kagan, Op. cit.

11 Guthe, Op. cit., 451.

12 Kagan, Op. cit.

13 Guthe, Op. cit.

14 Anon, "Doctors warn of increasing penicillin peril, some are susceptible to shock, death," *Chicago Daily Tribune* (May 8, 1953) 22.

15 V.A. Drill, *Pharmacology in Medicine: A Collaborative Textbook* (New York, Toronto, London) 1954. Quoted by Guthe, Op. cit.

16 A. Olszewski, et al., "Isolation and characterization of proteic allergens in refined peanut oil," *Clin Exp Allergy*, 28, 7 (July, 1998): 850-9. "In conclusion, we have demonstrated the presence of allergenic proteins in crude and refined peanut oil. These proteins are the same size as two allergens previously described in peanut protein extracts."

17 The Threshold Working Group, *Approaches to establish thresholds for major food allergens and for gluten in food* (FDA, March 2006). http://www.fda.gov/Food/LabelingNutrition/FoodAllergensLabeling/GuidanceComplianceRegulatoryInformation/ucm106108.htm

18 J.B. Greig & Joint FAO/WHO Expert Committee on Food Additives, "Potential allergenicity of refined food products, peanut oils and soya bean oils," *WHO Food Additive Series: 44* (Geneva, WHO, International Program on Chemical Safety, 2000) 8. http://www.inchem.org/documents/jecfa/jecmono/v44jec11.htm

19 D.A. Moneret-Vautrin, et al., "Risk of milk formulas containing peanut oil contaminated with peanut allergens in infants with atopic dermatitis," *Pediatr Allergy Immunol*, 5, 3(1994): 184-188.

20 G. De Montis, et al., "Sensitization to peanut and vitamin D oily preparations," *Lancet*, 341 (1993): 1411.

21 US Patent 3,696,189, Oct. 3, 1972.

22 O. Kayser, H. Rainer, *Pharmaceutical biotechnology*, (Wiley-VCH, 2004) 27.

23 A.E. Humphrey, F.H. Deindoerfer, "Microbiological Process Report," *Fermentation Process Review* (1960) 369. http://aem.asm.org/cgi/reprint/10/4/359.pdf

24 F. Scott Smyth, "Asthma in Children, Round Table Discussioin," Pediatrics, 2, 1 (July 1948): 119-131.

25 R. C. Harris, "The Treatment of Tetanus: Report of Two Cases with Critical Comment on New Therapeutic Resources," *Pediatrics*, 2 (Aug., 1948): 175-185.

26 A. Cantani, "Anaphylaxis from peanut oil in infant feedings and medications," *European Review of Medical and Pharmacological Sciences*, 2 (1998): 203-206.

27 D.A. Moneret-Vautrin, Op. cit.

28 Andrew Smith, *Peanuts, the illustrious history of the goober pea* (U. of Illnois Press, 2002) 65.

29 Ibid, 20.

30 Ibid, 67.

31 J. D. Stuart, "Peanuts and Patriotism," *Forum* 58 (Sept. 1917):375-80. In Smith, Op. cit., 205.

32 Smith, Op. cit., 100.

33 CDC, *National Occupational Exposure Survey (1981-1983)*. At greatest risk for hazardous exposure to peanut oil in the early 80s were veterinarians closely followed by telephone installers and repairers. http://www.cdc.gov/noes/noes2/a1216occ.html

34 Smith, Op. cit., 93.

35 Ibid, 102.

36 Ibid, 104.

37 Jane Holt, "News of Food; Peanut Crop, Worth $200,000,000 to South, Moving to Retail Stores in Various Forms," *New York Times*, (Sat. Nov. 11, 1944) 16.

38 Henry Lesesne, "Peanut Industry is Seeking Substitutes for War Uses, Report from the South," *St. Petersburg Times, Florida*, (Sept. 24, 1945) 2.

39 Jane Holt, "News of Food; Latest Shortage Looms in Peanut Supply for Civilians With a 50% Cut Forecast", *NY Times* (Sat. Jan. 6, 1945) 14.

40 Alfred Stefferud, "Big business in a nutshell," *New York Times Sunday Magazine* (Nov. 9, 1947) SM39.

41 Smith, 104. "$10,000,000 worth of peanuts were sold last year by Mssrs. Obici and Peruzzi, who own Planters Nut and Chocolate Co.," *Fortune* (April 1938) 80. Quoted by Smith, Op. cit., 55.

42 R.B. Borges, "Trade and the political economy of agricultural policy: the case of the United States Peanut Program," *Journal of Agriculture and Applied Economics*, 27, 2 (Dec., 1995): 595-612. http://ageconsearch.umn.edu/bitstream/15267/1/27020595.pdf The Agricultural Act of 1949 established acreage allotments for peanuts thus limiting the total amount of peanuts produced. Prior to 1978, all peanuts from these allotments were guaranteed a support price. These were quota peanuts. With technology more was grown on less land. For example, in 1950 allotment was 2,200,000 acres producing 2 billion pounds of peanuts. In 1981 allotment was 1,739 and production was nearly 4 billion pounds. Additional surplus quota peanuts were allowed but certain rules and different prices apply.

43 A.P. Black, "A new diagnostic method in allergic disease," *Pediatrics*, 17 (May 1956): 716-724. S. Goldman, et al, "Milk Allergy," Pediatrics, 32 (Sept. 1963): 425-443; and W.G. Crook, et al, "Systemic Manifestations due to allergy: Report on Fifty Patients," *Pediatrics*, 27 (May, 1961): 790-799. Both articles observe an increase in peanut and food allergy in children.

44 Smith, Op. cit., 208.

45 Borges, opt cit. NAFTA (1994), GATT (1995) and the US-Canada Free Trade Agreement (1989) have complicated the market and threatened to remove import barriers. These fears were unfounded since the 1995 Farm Bill continued subsidy for the farmers.

46 S.M. Fletcher, "Snack Peanuts Purchase Pattern," *Journal of Agricultural and Applied Economics*, 34, 1 (April, 2002).

47 E. Foko, *Transforming Mature Industries into Growth Industries: the Case of US Peanuts* (Kansas State U., 2008, master of Agribusiness) 10.

48 Stacy V. Jones, "Peanut Oil used in New Vaccine; product patented for Merck Said to Extend Immunity", *The New York Times, Business Financial Section* (Sept. 19, 1964) 31. Also reported in "Longer Life Vaccines," *The Age* (Monday, Dec. 7, 1964) 9.

49 United States Patent Office, 3,149,036, Sept. 15, 1964.

50 US Patent 3,149,036, Sept. 15, 1964.

51 Stacy V. Jones, opt cit.

52 Anon, "Peanut Oil Additive Is Found to Improve Flu Shot's Potency," *New York Times*, (Nov. 11 1966) p.33.

53 Emulsifying A process for preparing a highly stable water-in-oil type emulsion consisting of (a) a disperse aqueous phase; (b) a continuous oil phase containing isomannide monooleate emulsifier and a non-hydrated physiologically acceptable fatty acid metal salt. A particular use of the invention is the preparation of an emulsion adjuvant vaccine, wherein the vaccine is incorporated in the aqueous phase.
The emulsion is prepared by mixing the aqueous and oil phases at a relatively low agitator speed, optionally cooling, increasing the speed of agitation to form an emulsion and optionally homogenizing the emulsion

54 R.W. Howell, A.B. Mackenzie, "A Comparative trial of oil-adjuvant and aqueous polyvalent influencza vaccines," *Brit. J. industry. Med.*, 21 (1964): 265.

55 H. Nelson, "Expert Raises hope for improved flu vaccine, new serum produces 64 times more antibodies in animal tests, doctor says," *Los Angeles Times* (April 14, 1969) A 25.

56 J.W.G. Smith, et al., "Response to influenza vaccine in adjuvant 65-4," *J. Hyg*, 74, 2 (April, 1974): 251-259; M.R. Hilleman, A.F. Woodhour AF, A. Friedman, A.H. Phelps, "Studies for safety of Adjuvant 65," *Ann. Allergy*, 30 (1972): 477–80; R.E. Weibel, A. McLean, A.F. Woodhour, A. Friedman, M.R. Hilleman, "Ten-year follow-up study for safety of Adjuvant 65 influenza vaccine in man," *Proc. Soc. Exp. Biol. Medical*, 143 (1973): 1053–6.

57 Hilleman supported the use of peanut oil adjuvant in other vaccines such as one for cancer. Quoted in R. Kotulak, "He wants to vaccinate your child against cancer," *Chicago Tribune* (Feb. 24, 1974) M24.

58 N. Petrovsky, J. Cesar Aguilar, "Vaccine Adjuvants: Current State and Future Trends," *Immunology and Cell Biology*, 82 (2004): 488-496.

59 M.R. Hilleman, et al., "Immunological Adjuvants, Report of a WHO Scientific Group", *World Health Organization Technical Report Series, No. 595* (Geneva, World Health Organisation, 1976) 9.

60 Ibid, 11.

61 The Threshold Working Group, *Approaches to establish thresholds for major food allergens and for guten in food* (FDA, March, 2006).

62 Derek Hobson, "The potential role of immunological adjuvants in influenza vaccines," *Postgraduate Medical Journal*, 49 (March, 1973): 180-184;

63 Ibid, 183.

64 Interview with Adjuvant 65 developer Dr. Maurice Hilleman in Anon, "Human Cancer Virus Vaccines," *Cancer Journal for Clinicians*, 24 (1974): 212-217.

65 L. Galambos, *Networks of Innovation, Vaccine Development at Merck, Sharp & Dohme, and Mulford, 1895-1995* (Cambridge University Press, 1995) 138. The original Adjuvant 65 (1964) U.S. Pat. No. 3,149,036 was followed by U.S. Pat. No. 3,983,228 published Sept. 28, 1976 and U.S. Pat. No. 4,069,313 published in1978. Inventors of both adjuvants were A.F. Woodhour and M.R. Hilleman with the patent assigned to Merck & Co., Inc. The 1978 adjuvant for influenza improved on the original Adjuvant 65 (3149036 patent) in that it could be used with "proteinaceous antigen". It had a longer shelflife and it used "pure materials" that withstood de-emulsification.

66 Galambos, opt cit,138.

67 Manmohan Singh (ed.), *Vaccine adjuvants and delivery systems*, (New Jersey, Wiley, 2007) 6.

68 N. Goto, et al., "Studies on the Toxicities of Aluminum Hydroxide and Calcium Phosphate as Immunological Adjuvants for Vaccines," *Vaccine*, 11 (1993): 914–918; N.R. Butler, et al., "Advantages of aluminium hydroxide adsorbed combined diphtheria, tetanus, and pertussis vaccines for the immunization of infants," *British Medical Journal*, 1 1969): 663–666; F.M. Audibert, L.D. Lise, "Adjuvants: current status, clinical perspectives and future prospects.," Immunol Today, 14 (1993): 281–284; R. Bomford, "Aluminium salts: perspectives in their use as adjuvants", *Immunological Adjuvants and Vaccines* (New York: Plenum Press, 1989) 35–41; N. Petrovsky, Op. cit.

69 R.K. Gupta, et al., "Adjuvants - a balance between toxicity and adjuvanticity," *Vaccine*, 11, 4 (1993).

70 Research into the risks of vaccines is inadequate, according to two comprehensive reports on vaccines by the U.S. Institute of Medicine http://www.iom.edu in 1991 and 1994. The emerging nightmare scenario of inverse or reverse anaphylaxis describes an anaphylactic reaction not to an allergen or antigen (virus, bacteria) but to an antibody.

71 N. Petrovsky, J.C. Aguilar, "Vaccine Adjuvants: Current state and future trends*," Immunology and Cell Biology*, 82 (2004): 488-496.

72 R. Edelman, "Vaccine adjuvants," *Rev Infect Dis*, 2, 3 (1980). 370-383.

73 Petrovsky, Op. cit., 488.

74 D.E.S. Stewart-Tull, "Harmful and Beneficial Activities of Immunological Adjuvants," *Vaccine Adjuvants: Preparation Methods and Research Protocols*, (Humana Press, New Jersey, 2000) 30.

75 J.A. Reynolds, et al., "Adjuvant activity of a novel metabolizable lipid emulsion with inactivated viral vaccines," *Infect Immun.*, 28, 3 (June, 1980): 937-943.

76 http://www.patentstorm.us/patents/6299884/description.html; http://www.wipo.int/pctdb/en/wo.jsp?IA=WO2003018051&DISPLAY=DESC; US Patent 5679356; United States Patent 7361352

77 P. Gecher (ed.), *Encyclopedia of Emulsion Technology: Applications* (Marcel Dekker, 1985) 191.

78 A.C. Allison, N.E. Byars, "Immunologic adjuvants: general properties, and side-effects," *Mol Immunol.*, 28, 3 (March, 1991): 279–84.

79 K. Pollard, *Autoantibodies and Autoimmunity* (Wiley-VDH, 2006) 54.

80 Stewart-Tull, Op. cit., 29.

81 Val Brickates Kennedy, "BioSante: Promise for bird-flu drug," *MarketWatch* (April 24, 2006).

82 M. Khodoun, et al., "Peanuts can contribute to anaphylactic shock by activating complement," *J Allergy Clin Immunol.*, 123, 2 (Feb., 2009): 333-351.

83 S.J. Maleki, et al., "Structure of the Major Peanut Allergen Ara h 1 May Protect IgE-"Binding Epitopes from Degradation," J. Immunol., 1,164 (11 (June, 2000): 5844-9.

84 Wendy Harris, "Abnormal Response to Normal Things," *Professionally Speaking Magazine, Ontario College of Teachers* (Sept. 2000).

85 Institute of Medicine, Committee on Issues and Priorities for New Vaccine Development, *Vaccine Supply and Innovation* (Washington, DC, National Academy Press, 1985) 10.

86 Anon, "Vaccination Litigation," *Trial Lawyers Inc., Health Care* (2005). http://www.triallawyersinc.com/healthcare/hc04.html#notes

87 Regarding the 1976 "pandemic" see A.M. Silverstein, *Pure Politics and Impure Science* (Johns Hopkins U. Press, 1981). See also A.D. Langmuir, et al., "An epidemiologic and Clinical Evaluation of Guillan-Barre Syndrome Reported in Association with the Administration of Swine Influenza Vaccines," *American Journal of Epidemiology*, 119, 6 (1984): 841-79.

88 Anon, *Vaccination Litigation*, Trial Lawyers, Inc. (2005) cites E. W. Kitch, *Vaccines and Product Liability: A Case of Contagious Litigation*, Regulation, (May/June 1985) 13.

89 Ibid. "Statement of Robert B. Johnson, president, Lederle Laboratories Division, American Cyanamid, House Subcommittee on Health and the Environment," *Vaccine Injury Compensation* (Sept. 10, 1984).

90 Galambos, Op. cit., 148.

91 Institute of Medicine, Committee on Issues and Priorities for New Vaccine Development, *Vaccine Supply and Innovation* (Washington, DC., National Academy Press, 1985). The National Institute of Allergy and Infectious Diseases (NIAID, part of the National Institute of Health) proposed an acceleration program for new vaccines. The Dept. of Health and Human Services would conduct the program. The steering committee of the Dept. of Health and Human Services launched a study of the problem. Three studies emerged in 1985 produced by the Institute of Medicine.

92 Eligible claims are for reactions must have lasted more than 6 months after the vaccine was given, resulted in hospital stay, surgery or death. The Vaccine Adverse Event Reporting System cosponsored by the FDA and the CDC established in 1990 is not linked to the VICP.

93 Galambos, Op. cit., 178.

94 Statistical Abstracts of the United States, *Percent of Children Immunized Against Specific Diseases, by Age Group: 1980 to 1985*. See also F.T. Cutts, et al., "Causes of Low Preschool Immunization Coverage in the United States," *Annual Review of Public Health*, 13 (May, 1992): 385-398.

95 Anon, "Improving the Chances of Survival," *The World Health Report, Chapter 6* (WHO, 2005) http://www.who.int/whr/2005/chapter6/en/index1.html

96 IOM, *The Children's Vaccine Initiative: achieving the Vision* (Washington, The National Academies Press, 1993).

97 Institute of Medicine, "Committee on Issues and Priorities for New Vaccine Development", *New Vaccine Development: Establishing Priorities, 1* (Washington DC, 1985).

98 Galambos, Op. cit., 177.

99 US patent application 06/395743 filed Jan. 6, 1982.

100 A.L. Smith, "Antibiotics and Invasive Haemophilus Influenzae," *New England Journal of Medicine*, 294, 24 (1976): 1329-31.

101 E.O. Mason, et al., "Serotype and ampicillin susceptibility of Haemophilus Influenzae causing system infections in children: 3 years of experience," *Journal of Clinical Microbiology*, 15, 4 (April, 1982): 543-546.

102 http://www.merck.com/product/usa/pi_circulars/p/pedvax_hib/pedvax_pi.pdf

103 K.C. Schoendort, "National trends in Haemophilus influenzae meningitis mortality and hospitalization among children, 1980 through 1991," *Pediatrics*, 93, 4 (April, 1994): 663-8.

104 The license was in part based on a clinical trial in North Carolina (1977) that involved 16,00 children aged two months to five years. In another Finnish trial 48,977 children three months to five years were injected with the vaccine. Folllow up studies indicated that it was ineffective and had resulted in adverse reactions. It was also noted that it actually increased incidence of the disease right after immunization, in less than seven days.

105 K.R. Stratton, et al., (eds.) IOM, "Haemophius influenzae Type b Vaccines, Background and History", *Adverse Events Associated with Childhood Vaccines* (Washington, National Academies Press, 1994) 236.

106 D. Goldblatt, "Recent developments in bacterial conjugate vaccines," *J Med Micro.*, 47 (1998): 563-7.

107 R.S. Daum, et al, "Decline in serum antibody to the capsule of Haemophilus influenzae type b in the immediate postimmunization period." J Pediatr., 114 (1989): 742-747.

108 K.R. Stratton, et al., (eds.) IOM, "Causality and Evidence," Op. cit., 238.

109 Ibid, 237

110 FDA summary for Basis of Approval for ActHIB has important information blacked out including induction of higher levels of Ig_ relative to Ig_" http://www.fda.gov/downloads/BiologicsBloodVaccines/Vaccines/ApprovedProducts/UCM109864.pdf

111 Ibid, 237.

112 Ibid.

113 Viera Scheibner, *Vaccination* (Australia, McPherson's, 1993) 130.

114 Julie Milstien, B. Candries, "Economics of vaccine development and implementation: changes over he past 20 years," WHO (Geneva, 1998)

115 M.T. Jelonek, et al, "Comparison of naturally acquired and vaccine-induced antibodies to Haemophilus influenzae type b capsular polysaccharide," *Infection and Immunity*, 61, 12 (Dec., 1993): 5345-5350

116 G. Rothrock, et al., "Haemophilus influenzae Invasive Disease Among Children Aged <5 Years—California, 1990-1996," *JAMA,* 280 (1998):1130-1131.

117 Anon, "Current Trends Vaccination Coverage of 2-Year-Old Children – United States, 1993," *MMWR, CDC*, 43, 39 (Oct. 7, 1994): 705-709. Vaccination coverage increased for three vaccines from 1992 to 1993: for three or more doses of Hib, from 28.0% to 49.9%; for three or more doses of poliomyelitis vaccine, from 72.4% to 78.4%; and for three or more doses of DPT/diphtheria and tetanus toxoids (DT), from 83.0% to 87.2%. Coverage with measles-containing vaccine decreased from 82.5% to 80.8%. Among 19-35-month-olds, 12.7% had received three or more doses of Hep B. From 1992 to 1993, the proportion of children who had received a combined series of four or more doses of DPT/DT, three or more doses of polio vaccine, and one dose of MMR increased from 55.3% to 64.8%, primarily because of increased coverage with the fourth DPT/DT dose (from 59.0% to 71.1%). At the start of 1994, Hib coverage was a record high of 70.6% and and hepatitis B 25.5%.

118 *Disease prevention through vaccine development and immunization, The U.S. National Vaccine Plan – 1994*, Dept. of Health and Human Services, Public Health Service, National Vaccine Program Office (1994).

119 IOM, *Calling the Shots: Immunization Finance Policies and Practices* (Washington, National Academy Press, 2000) 252.

120 Gary Walsh, *Biopharmaceuticals* (John Wiley and Sons, 2003).

121 Anon, "Changes to the Australian Standard Vaccination Schedule (1992-2005)," *Vaccine Preventable Diseases and Vaccination Coverage in Australia, 2003 to 2005*, Appendix 4, Department of Health and Ageing, Australian Government. http://www.health.gov.au

122 D.M. Salisbury, et al., "Vaccine programmes and policies," *British Medical Bulletin*, 62 (2002): 201-211 (2002). http://bmb.oxfordjournals.org/cgi/content/full/62/1/201

123 http://www.healthheritageresearch.com/Pertussis/Pertussis-Vaccine-History-CAN-ex-ho.pdf

124 Advisory Committee on Immunization Practices, "Combined vaccines for childhood immunization," *Morbidity and Mortality Weekly Report (MMWR)CDC*, 48, RR05 (May 14, 1999: 1-15

125 M.J. Corbel, "Control testing of combined vaccines: A consideration of potential problems and approaches," *Biologicals*, 22 (1994):353-60; J. Eskola, et al., "Randomized trial of the effect of co-administration with acellular pertussis DPT vaccine on immunogenicity of Haemophilus influenzae type b conjugate vaccine," *Lancet*, 348 (1996): 1688-92.

126 P.A. Di Sant-Agnese, "Combined immunization against diphtheria, tetanus and pertussis in newborn infants," *Pediatrics*, 3, 3 (March, 1949): 333-344.

127 M.A. Valdes-Dapena, "Sudden and unexpected death in infancy: a review of the world literature 1954-1966," Pediatrics, 39, 1 (Jan. 1967): 123-138. This article reviewed the issue sudden infant death syndrome, SIDS. Commenting on the up to 25,000 infant deaths each year, the author professed to be "woefully ignorant". A connection was soon made between these deaths and vaccination: W.C. Torch, "Diptheria-pertussis-tetanus (DPT) immunization: A potential cause of the sudden infant death syndrome (SIDS), *Neurology*, 32, 4(1982): 2. In the mid 1970's Japan raised their vaccination age from two months to two years resulting in a significant drop in incidence of SIDS.

128 R. Dagan, "Reduced response to multiple vaccines sharing common protein epitopes that are administered simultaneously to infants," *Infect Immun.*, 66, 5(May, 1998):2093-8.

129 A.M. Barnam, S.L. Lukacs, "Food Allergy Among U.S. Children: Trends in Prevalence and Hospitalizations," *National Centre for Health Statistics, CDC* (Oct. 22, 2008). This trend has continued. Four in every 100 US children has severe food allergy.

130 S.Allan Bock, et al, "Fatalities due to anaphylactic reactions to food," *Journal of Allergy and Clinical Immun.*, 107, 1 (Jan., 2001): 191-93.

131 S.H. Sicherer, et al., "Prevalence of peanut and tree nut allergy in the United States determined by means of a random digit dial telephone survey: a 5-year follow up study," *JACI*, 112, 6 (Dec. 2003): 1203-1207.

PART 3: Peanut Allergy at the Crossover Point

CHAPTER 6: Absorbing the Costs

1 A.W. Taylor-Robinson, "Multiple vaccination effects on atopy," *Allergy*, 54 (1999): 398-399.

2 http://www.cdc.gov/vaccines/pubs/pinkbook/downloads/appendices/B/excipient-table-2.pdf

3 R.K. Gupta, "Adjuvants, a balance between toxicity and adjuvanticity," *Vaccine*, 11, 3 (Jan., 1993): 293-306.

4 R.K. Gupta, G.R. Siber, "Adjuvants for human vaccines—current status, problems and future prospects," *Vaccine*, 13, 14 (1995): 1263-1276.

5 N. Petrovsky, et al., "New-Age Vaccine Adjuvants: Friend or Foe?" *Biopharm International* (August 2, 2007): 6. http://biopharminternational.findpharma.com

6 D.A. Salmon, et al., "Enhancing public confidence in vaccines through independent oversight of postlicensure vaccine safety," *Am J Public Health*, 94, 6 (June, 2004): 947-950.

7 P.H. Dennehy, "Active Immunization in the United States: Developments over the Past Decade," *Clin Microbiol Rev.*, 14, 4 (Oct., 2001): 872-908. http://ukpmc.ac.uk/articlerender.cgi?artid=127650

8 A.W. Taylor-Robinson, Op. cit.

9 K. Stratton, et al., IOM, *Immunization Safety Review: Multiple immunizations and immune dysfunction* (Washington, National Academy Press, 2002) 36.

10 Various, "Workshop on Aluminum in Vaccines", *Transcript, Dept. of Health and Human Services, National Vaccine Program Office and jointly sponsored by Task Force for Child Survival and Development Transcript of meeting held at the Caribe Hilton International Hotel, San Juan, Puerto Rico*, 2 (May 11, 2000): 105. This meeting was attended by representative experts from the WHO, industry, government, academia and interested individuals.

11 Ibid, 78.

12 Ibid, 191.

13 Stanley Hem, "Absorption andElimination of Aluminum-containing adjuvants," from "Workshop on Aluminum in Vaccines", Op. cit.

14 F. Andre, et al., "Gelatin prepared from tuna skin: a risk factor for fish allergy or sensitization?" *Immunology*, 130, 1, (2003).

15 T. Nakayama, T. Kumagai, "Gelatin Allergy," *Pediatrics*, 113, 1, (Jan., 2004): 170-171.

16 T. Nakayama, et al., "A clinical analysis of gelatin allergy and determination of its causal relationship to the previous administration of gelatin-containing acellular pertussis vaccine combined with diphtheria and tetanus toxoids," *J Allergy Clin Immunol.*,103, 1 (1999): 321-5; R. Wahl, D.

Kleinhans, "IgE-mediated allergic reactions to fruit gums and investigation of cross-reactivity between gelatine and modified gelatine-containing products," *Clin Exp Allergy*,19, 1 (1989): 77-80; M. Sakaguchi, et al., "Food allergy to gelatin in children with systemic immediate-type reactions, including anaphylaxis, to vaccine," *J Allergy Clin Immunol.*, 98,1 (1996):1058-61; J.M. Kelso, et al., "Anaphylaxis to measles, mumps, and rubella vaccine mediated by IgE to gelatin," *J Allergy Clin Immunol.*, 91, 4 (1993): 867-72; S. Singer S, et al., "Urticaria following varicella vaccine associated with gelatin allergy," *Vaccine*, 17, 4 (1999): 3279.

17 T. Nakayama, C. Aizawa, "Change in gelatin content of vaccines associated with reduction in reports of allergic reactions," *J Allergy Clin Immunol.*,106 (2000): 591–592.

18 V. Pool, et al., "Prevalence of Anti-gelatin IgE antibodies in people with anaphylaxis after measles-mump-rubella vaccine in the United States," *Pediatrics*, 110, 6 (Dec. 2002): e71.

19 A. Patja, et al., "Allergic Reaction to Measles-Mumps-Rubella Vaccination," *Pediatrics*, 107, 2 (Feb. 2001): e27.

20 http://www.patentstorm.us/patents/6299884/description.html
US Patent 5679356. United States Patent 7361352

21 L. Heller, "Peanut oil production doubles with new US Golden Peanut refiner," *Food Navigator USA, Financial & Industry* (Jan. 17, 2007). http://www.foodnavigator-usa.com/Financial-Industry/Peanut-oil-production-doubles-with-new-US-Golden-Peanut-refinery

22 D.A. Moneret Vautrin, et al., "Risks of milk formulas containing peanut oil contaminated with peanut allergens in infants with atopic dermatitis," *Pediatric Allergy and Immunology*, 5, 3 (Dec., 1993): 184-188.

23 A. Cantani, "Anaphylaxis from peanut oil in infant feedings and medications," *European Review of Medical and Pharmacological Sciences*, 2 (1998): 203-206.

24 A. Olszewski, et al., "Isolation and characterization of proteic allergens in refined peanut oil," *Clin Exp Allergy*, 28, 7 (July, 1998): 850-9.

25 Threshold Working Group, "Approaches to Establish Thresholds for Major Food Allergens and for Gluten in Food," *Food Allergens Labeling*, U.S. Food and Drug Administration (March 2006).

26 Anon, "Opinion of the Scientific Panel on Dietetic Products, Nutritionand Allergies on a request from the Commission related to a notification fro FEDIOL and IMACE on fully refined peanut oil and fat pursuant to Article 6, paragraph 11 of Directive 2000/13/EC," *The EFSA Journal*, 133 (Oct. 19, 2004): 1-9.

27 J.B. Greig & Joint FAO/WHO Expert Committee on Food Additives, "Potential allergenicity of refined food products, peanut oils and soya bean oils*," WHO Food Additive Series, International Program on Chemical Safety*, 44 (2000): 8. http://www.inchem.org/documents/jecfa/jecmono/v44jec11.htm

28 Anon, "Listing of Food Additive Status", *Food Additives*, U.S. Food and Drug Administration (March, 2009).

29 Threshold Working Group, "Approaches to Establish Thresholds for Major Food Allergens and for Gluten in Food," *Food Allergens Labeling*, U.S. Food and Drug Administration (March 2006).

30 Anon, "Guidelines, Medicinal products for human use, safety, environment and information, Excipients in the label and package leaflet of medicinal products for human use," *European Commission*, 3B (Brussels, July 2003) 5.
http://www.emea.europa.eu/pdfs/human/productinfo/3bc7a_200307en.pdf

31 George Wade, EMEA, "Query Response: Arachis Oil: Inquiry No. 11-273," November 20, 2009. This is an email query response.

32 J. Swarbrick, J.C. Boylan (eds.), *Encyclopedia of pharmaceutical technology*, 19 (Basel, Marcel Dekker, 2000) 290.

33 Jean Mayer, "Better Labeling laws are needed," *Pittsburgh Post-Gazette* (June 5, 1972) 12.

34 G. Lack, et al., "Avon Longitudinal Study of Parents and Children Study Team. Factors associated with the development of peanut allergy in childhood. *N Engl J Med.*, 348 (2003): 977-85.

35 A. Olszewski, et al., "Isolation and characterization of proteic allergens in refined peanut oil," *Clin Exp Allergy*, 28, 7 (July, 1998): 850-9.

36 M. Khodoun, et al., "Peanuts can contribute to anaphylactic shock by activating complement," *J Allergy Clin Immunol.*, 123, 2 (Feb., 2009): 333-351.

37 S.J. Maleki, et al. "Structure of the Major Peanut Allergen Ara h 1 May Protect IgE-"Binding Epitopes from Degradation," *J. Immunol.*, 164, 11 (June, 2000): 5844-9.

38 I.N. Glaspole, et al., "Anaphylaxis to lemon soap: citrus seed and peanut allergen cross-reactivity," *Ann Allergy Asthma Immunol,*, 98, 3 (March, 2007): 286-9.

39 R. Ellis, D. Granoff (ed), *Development and clinical uses of haemophilus b conjugate vaccines* (New York, Marcel Dekker, 1994) 120.

40 J. W. Coleman, M. Blanca, "Mechanisms of drug allergy", *Immunology Today*, 19, 5 (May 1998): 196-198; A. Cantani, *Pediatric allergy, asthma and immunology*, (Germany, Springer, 2008) 1150; A.L. Schocket (ed.), *Clinical management of uticaria and anaphylaxis*, (US, Marcel Dekker, Inc., 1993) 120.

41 M. Frieri, B. Kettelhut (eds.), *Food Hypersensitivity and adverse reactions: a practical guide for diagnosis Clinical Allergy and Immunology* (CRC Press, 1999) 84.

42 S. D. Kelleher, et al. "Functional Chicken Muslcle Protein Isolates…" *53rd Annual Reciprocal Meat Conference, American Meat Science Association* (2000) www.meatscience.org Beef serum albumin and muscle protein (BSA and BGG) has a molecular weight of between 17 and 66 kD; albumin in egg 45 kD.

43 P.A. Gulig, E.J. Hansen, "Coprecipitation of lipopolysaccharide and the 39,000-molecular-weight major outer membrane protein of Haemophilus influenzae type by by lipopolysaccharide-directed monoclonal antibody," *Infect Immun.*, 49, 3 (Sept., 1985): 819-827.

44 A. Kimura, et al., "A minor high-molecular-weight outer membrane protein of Haemophilus influenzae type by is a protective antigen," *Infect Immun.*, 47, 1 (Jan., 1985): 253-259.

45 R. Fischer, et al., "Oral and Nasal Sensitization Promote distinct immune responses and reactivity in a mouse model of peanut allergy," *American Journal of Pathology*, 167 (2005): 1621-1630; F. van Wijk, et al., "The CD28/CTLA-4-B7 signaling pathway is involved in both allergic sensitization ad tolerance induction to orally administered peanut proteins," *The Journal of Immunology*,178 (2007): 6894-6900.

46 A.van den Biggelaar, et al., "Neonatal pneumococcal conjugate vaccine immunization primes T cells for preferential Th2 cytokine expression: a randomized controlled trial in Papua New Guinea," *Vaccine*, 27, 9 (Feb., 2009): 1340-1347.

47 D.C. Wilson, et al., "The Window of opportunity: pre-pregnancy to 24 months of age, induction of antigen-specific immunity in human neonates and infants*," Nestle Nutrition Workshop, Senior Pediatric Program*, 61 (2008): 183-95.

48 M.R. Nelson, et al., Anaphylaxis complicating routine childhood immunization: hemophilus influenza b conjugated vaccine," *Pediatric Asthma, Allergy & Immunology*, 14, 4 (Dec., 2000): 315-321.

49 R. Schneerson, et al., "Preparation, characterization, and immunogenicity of haemophilus influenzae type b polysaccharide-protein conjugates," *Journal of Experimental Medicine*, 152 (1980): 361-375.

50 A. Schuster, et al. "Does pertussis infection induce manifestation of allergy?" *Journal of Molecular Medicine*, 71, 3 (March 1992): 208-213.

51 A. Dannemann, et al., "Specific IgE and IgG4 immune respones to tetanus and diphtheria toxoid in atopic and non-atopic children during the first two years of life," *International Archives of Allergy and Immunology*, 111, 3 (1996): 262-267.

52 J. Nagel, et al., "IgE synthesis in man, development of specific IgE antibodies after immunization with tetanus-diphtheria (Td) toxoids," *J Immunol.*, 118, 1 (Jan., 1977): 334-41.

53 A. Mark, et al., "Immuoglobulin E respones to diphtheria and tetanus toxoids after booster with aluminium absorbed and fluid DT-vaccines," *Vaccine*,13, 7(May,1995): 669-73.

54 D. G. Marsh, M.N. Blumenthal," *Genetic and Enviornmental Factors in Clinical Allergy*, (University of Minnesota Press, 1990) 92

55 U. Kosecka, et al. "Pertussis adjuvant prolongs intestinal hypersensitivity*," Int Arch Allergy Immunol.*, 119, 3 (July, 1999): 205-11.

56 M. Flora Martin-Munoz, "Anaphylactic reaction to diphtheria-tetanus vaccine in a child: specific IgE IgG determinations and cross-reactivity studies," *Vaccine*, 20, 27-28 (Sept. 2002): 3409-3412.

57 C. Mayorga, et al., "Immediate allergy to tetanus toxoid vaccine: determination of immunoglobulin E and immunoglobulin G antibodies to allergenic proteins," *Ann Allergy Asthma Immunol.*, 90, 2 (Feb., 2003): 238-43

58 B. Bellioni Businco, et al., "Allergy to tetanus toxoid vaccine," *Allergy*, 56, 7 (2001): 701-2

59 S. Hadenskog, "Immunoglobulin E Response to Pertussis Toxin in Whooping Cough and after Immunization with a Whole-Cell and an Acellular Pertussis Vaccine," *Int Arch Allergy and Immunology*, 89 (1989):156-161.

60 Kosecka, Op. cit.

61 Xiu-Min Li, et al., "Engineered Recombinant peanut protein and heat –killed Listeria monocytogenes co-administration protects against peanut-induced anaphylaxis," *The Journal of Immunology*, 170 (2003): 3289-3295.

62 N.O. Eghafona, "Immune responses following cocktails of inactivated measles vaccine and Arachis hypogaea L. (ground nut) or Cocos nucifera L. (coconut) oils adjuvant," *Vaccine*, 17-18, 14 (Dec., 1996): 1703-6.

63 F. Audibert, L. Chedid, "Adjuvant disease induced by mycobacteria, determinants of arthritogenicity," *Agents Actions*, 1-3, 6 (Feb., 1976): 75-85.

64 Xiu-min Li, et al., "Strain-dependent induction of allergic sensitization caused by peanut allergen DNA immunization in Mice," *The Journal of Immunology*, 162 (1999): 3045-3052.

65 K. Redhead, et al., "Combination of DPT and Haemophilus influenzae type b conjugate vaccines can affect laboratory evaluation of potency and immunogenicity," Biologicals, 22, 4 (Dec., 1994): 339-45

66 Petrovsky, Op. cit., 188.

67 D.E.S. Stewart-Tull, "Harmful and Beneficial Activities of Immunological Adjuvants," *Vaccine Adjuvants: Preparation Methods and Research Protocols*, (Humana Press, New Jersey, 2000) 30.

68 Y.S. Lee, et al., "Invasive Haemophilus influenzae type b infections in Singapore children: a hospital-based study," *Journal of Paediatrics and Child Health*, 36, 2 (2000): 125-127.

69 F.S. Lim, et al., "Primary vaccination of infants against hepatitis B can be completed using a combined hexavalent diphtheria-tetanus-acellular pertussis-hepatitis B-inactivated poliomyelitis-Haemophilus influenzae type B vaccine," *Ann Acad Med Singapore*, 36, 10 (Oct., 2007): 801-6.

70 D.J. Hill, et al., "The frequency of food allergy in Australia and Asia," *Environmental Toxicology and Pharmacology*, 4, 1-2(Nov., 1997) : 101-110; L. Shek Pei-Chi, Asst. Prof. Dept. of Pediatrics, National University of Singapore, "Food Allergy in Children" (Jan., 2005). This article is on-line at NUS http://www.med.nus.edu.sg/paed/academic/AP_food_allergy.htm

71 L. Shek Pei-Chi, Op. cit.

72 C. Crooks, et al., "The changing epidemiology of food allergy, implications for New Zealand," *The New Zealand Medical Journal*, 121, 1271 (April 4, 2008).

73 Malaria Vaccine, Decision-Making Framework, "Overview of National Immunization Program in Ghana," undated. Online at www.malvacdecsion.net/ http://www.malvacdecision.net/pdfs/Overview%20of%20Immunization%20in%20Ghana%205-12-06.pdf Despite the documented sensitivity to peanut, these children were not actively reactive to the food. An important element in this case appeared to have been the helminths. As discussed in the Helminth Hypothesis, these intestinal worms render those infected hyporeactive. No one knows at what level they confer allergy suppression but it appeared that helminths were masking the peanut allergy.

74 E.N.C. Mills, et al., "The prevalence, cost and basis of food allergy across Europe," *Allergy*, 62, 7 (July, 2007): 717-722.

75 A.E. Platonov, et al., "Economic evaluation of Haemophilus influenzae type b vaccination in Moscow, Russian Federation," *Vaccine*, 24,13 (March, 2006): 2367-2376.

76 www.hibaction.org/resources/presentations/TechnicalHibVaccine.ppt

77 A. Kemp, "Severe peanut allergy in Australian children," *Med J of Australia*, 183, 5 (2005): 277; A.L. Ponsonby, et al., "A prospective study of the association between home gas appliance use during infancy and subsequent dust mite sensitization and lung function in childhood," *Clin Exp Allergy*, 31 (2001):1544-1552

78 Linda Smith, "Nut allergies skyrocket," *The Mercury, The Voice of Tasmania* (Feb. 26, 2009).

79 Ibid.

80 M.R. Kilmartin, et al., ""Immunisation of babies, the mothers' perspective," *Aust Fam Physician*, 27 (Jan., 1998): S11-4.

81 Anon, "Changes to the Australian Standard Vaccination Schedule (1992-2005)," *Communicable Diseases Intelligence*, 31 (June 2007). In 1995 the DPT vaccination replaced the CDT vaccination (combined diphtheria tetanus) for children prior to school entry. In 1992, the MMR vaccine was introduced. In 1993, Hib was introduced. Combined DPTa-hepB-IPV-Hib was introduced in 2001 and DPTa-IPV-Hib (PRP-T) in Nov. 2005. In 2001, the combined 5 in 1 vaccine with Hib was

approved for use in Australia. http://www.health.gov.au/internet/main/publishing.nsf/Content/cda-cdi31suppl.htm~cda-cdi31suppl-apx4.htm

82 http://www.health.gov.au/internet/main/publishing.nsf/Content/cda-cdi28suppl2d.htm Anon, "Vaccine Preventable Diseases and Vaccination Coverage in Australia, 2001 to 2002 - Vaccination Coverage," *Communicable Diseases Intelligence*, 28, 2 (Dec., 2004)

83 Anon, "Changes to the Australian Standard Vaccination Schedule (1992-2005), Communicable Diseases Intelligence, 31 (June 2007).
http://www.health.gov.au/internet/main/publishing.nsf/Content/cda-cdi31suppl.htm~cda-cdi31suppl-apx4.htm
84 Anon, "Vaccine Preventable Diseases and Vaccination Coverage in Australia, 2001 to 2002, Vaccination Coverage," *Communicable Diseases Intelligence*, 28, 2 (Dec. 2004).
http://www.health.gov.au/internet/main/publishing.nsf/Content/cda-cdi28suppl2d.htm

85 ACT is a self-governing state within New South Wales with the highest density population and smallest area at 2,358 km. Within it is the national capital of Canberra.
86 Linda Smith, Op. cit.
87 M. Kijakovic, et al., "The parent-reported prevalence and management of peanut and nut allergy in school children in the Australian Capital Territory," *Journal of Paediatrics and Child Health*, 45 (March, 2009); R.J. Mullins, "Characteristics of childhood peanut allergy in the Australian Capital Territory 1995 to 2007," *J Allergy and Clin Immunol.*, 123, 3 (March, 2009): 689-693. R.J. Mullins, "Paediatric food allergy trends in a community-based specialist allergy practice, 1995-2006," *Medical Journal of Australia*,186, 12 (2007): 618-621. Over 12 years, Mullins saw the demand for food allergy services increase 400% in his practice for children aged 0-5. Peanut, tree nut, egg and dairy were the common triggers. Mullins interpreted the dramatic increase in hospital admissions for anaphylaxis in Australia at twice that described in UK studies as as evidence of a food allergy "epidemic".
88 Anon, "Health Status: Protecting the health of our children," *Austrlian Social Trends, Australian Bureau of Statistics*, 41020 (June, 1997). http://www.abs.gov.au/
89 Profet, Op. cit., 36
90 K. Bock, *Healing the New Childhood Epidemics, Autism, ADHD, Asthma, and Allergies* (New York, Random House, 2007) 19.
91 Ibid.
92 T.D. Green, Op. cit.
93 S.H. Sicherer, et al., "Clinical features of acute allergic reactions to peanut and tree nuts in children," *Pediatrics*, 102, 1 (1998): e6
94 T.K. Vander Leek, et al., "The natural history of peanut allergy in young children and its association with serum peanut-specific IgE, *J Pediatr.*, 137 (2000): 749-755; H.S. Skolnik, et al., "The natural history of peanut allergy," *J. Allergy Clin Immunol.*, 107 (2001): 367-374.
95 Mullins, Op. cit., 4.
96 S. Sicherer, et al., "Prevalence of peanut and tree nut allergy in the United States determined by means of a random digit dial telephone survey: a 5 year follow up study," *Journal of Allergy and Clin Immunol.*, 112 (2003): 1203-1207.
97 S. Cave, "Testimony," Committee on Government Reform, U.S. House of Representatives (July 18, 2000). http://www.healing-arts.org/children/autismandmercurytestimony.htm

CHAPTER 7: Rationalizations

1 N. Petrovsky, et al., "New-Age Vaccine Adjuvants: Friend or Foe?" *Biopharm International* (August 2, 2007): 6. http://biopharminternational.findpharma.com
2 T. Nakayama, T. Kumagai, "Gelatin Allergy," *Pediatrics*, 113, 1, (Jan., 2004): 170-171.
3 Stuart Anderson, *Making Medicines: a brief history of pharmacy and pharmaceuticals* (Pharmaceutical Press, 2005) 156.
4 A.W. Taylor-Robinson, "Multiple vaccination effects on atopy," *Allergy*, 54 (1999): 398-399, (1999)
5 Charles Richet, *The Nobel Prize in Physiology or Medicine 1913, Nobel Lecture* (Dec. 11, 1913).
http://nobelprize.org/nobel_prizes/medicine/laureates/1913/richet-lecture.html

6 C. Anandan, A. Sheikh, "Preventing development of allergic disorders in children," *BMJ*, 333 (2006): 485.

7 *Scientific Review of Vaccine Safety Datalink Information*, Simpsonwood Retreat Center, Norcross Georgia (June 7-8, 2000). In attendance at this meeting called by the Center for Disease Control were the CDC's Advisory Committee on Immunization Practices (ACIP), American Academy of Pediatrics (AAP) and 48 other well regarded institutions as well as members from GlaxoSmithKline, Merck, Wyeth and Aventis Pasteur. Both transcript and report are available at www.autismhelpforyou.com

8 The report and transcript are discussed in Robert F. Kennedy Jr., "Deadly Immunity," *Salon.com* (June 16, 2005).

9 Anon, The Man Behind the Vaccine Mystery, *CBS Evening News* (Dec. 12, 2002). www.cbsnews.com

10 Various, *Scientific Review of Vaccine Safety Datalink Information*, Transcript of Meeting held at the Simpsonwood Retreat Center, Norcross Georgia (June 7-8, 2000) 248.

11 "Study Autism prevalence still up after Thimerosal removed from vaccines, New genetic link found," *American Academy of Family Physicians* (Jan. 16, 2008). http://www.aafp.org

12 Alice Park, "The Truth About Vaccines," *Time Magazine* (Canadian Edition, June 2, 2008) 34.

13 Tim Vawter vs. Federal government, presented to USDNY on July 31, 2009. http://www.safetylawsuits.com/prelim-injunction.html The injunction was filed simultaneous with WHO news that 1 billion doses of adjuvanted H1N1 swine flu vaccine containing Thimerosol had been sold to western countries according.

14 Anon, "Canada to order 50.4 million H1N1 vaccine doses," *CBC News*, Aug. 6, 2009. http://www.cbc.ca/health/story/2009/08/06/swine-flu-vaccine.html In Canada the government contract for 50.4 million doses costing $40 million was granted to Glaxo SmithKline which uses an "adjuvant advantage".

15 Val Brickates Kennedy, "BioSante: Promise for bird-flu drug," *MarketWatch* (April 24, 2006).

16 "Seasonal Ifluenza: the economics of vaccination," *Center for Prevention and Health Services* (Oct. 2006)

17 C.W. Shepard, et al.,"Cost-effectiveness of conjugate meningococcal vaccination strategies in the United States," *Pediatrics*, 115, 5 (May, 2005): 1220-1232.

18 Julie Milstien, B. Candries, "Economics of vaccine development and implementation: changes over he past 20 years," WHO (Geneva, 1998) http://www.who.int/immunization_supply/introduction/economics_vaccineproduction.pdf

19 Rep. Henry A. Waxman, "Analysis, pharmaceutical industry profits increase by over $8 billion after Medicare drug plan goes into effect," Report, Rep. Henry A. Waxman, Ranking Minority member, Committee on Government Reform, US House of Representatives, Sept. 2006 http://oversight.house.gov/documents/20060919115623-/0677.pdf

20 Annys Shin, "Food allergies trigger multibillion-dollar specialty market," *The Washington Post* (Sun., June 8, 2008). Online: http://www.washingtonpost.com/wp-dyn/content/article/2008/06/07/AR2008060702125.html

21 James Altucher, "Save the children (and make money)," *Wall Street Journal, Investing* (August 10, 2009) http://online.wsj.com/article/SB124992390387319939.html

22 Dr. Eugene Robin, "Letter to The First International Public Conference on Vaccination", *Mothering*, 86 (January/February 1998). Reprinted in http://www.mothering.com/health/first-international-public-conference-vaccination

APPENDIX

1 Daniel Boakye, "Infections and Food Allergy in Africa," Noguchi Memorial Institute for Medical Research http://ec.europa.eu; B.B. Obeng, et al., "Allergic sensitization and reported adverse reactiosn to food in Ghanaian school children: a nested case-control study," *Journal of Allergy and Clinical Immunology*, 123, 2 (Feb. 2009): S31.

2 G. Du Toit, et al., "Peanut allergy and peanut-specific IgG4 characteristics among Xhosan children in Cape Town," *J Allergy Clin Immunol.*, 119, 1 (Jan. 2007): S196. Malnourishment of children is a significant problem in Algeria for example where fat based spread fortified with nutrients is made

from dried lactoserum and peanut butter. Allergic reaction has not been a problem in the settings where the spread has been used by WHO a field trial in Algeria.

3 D.M. Lewis, General Practitioner Watford, UK letter in response to C. Anandan, A. Sheikh, "Preventing development of allergic disorders in children," British Medical Journal, 333 (2006): 485.

4 M. Kijakovic, et al., "The parent-reported prevalence and management of peanut and nut allergy in school children in the Australian Capital Territory," *Journal of Paediatrics and Child Health*, 45 (March, 2009):3; R.J. Mullins, "Paediatric food allergy trends in a community-based specialist allergy practice, 1995-2006," *Medical Journal of Australia*, 186, 12 (2007): 618-621. Over 12 years, Mullins saw the demand for food allergy services increase 400% in his practice for children aged 0-5. Peanut, tree nut, egg and dairy were the common triggers. Mullins interpreted the dramatic increase in hospital admissions for anaphylaxis in Australia at twice that described in UK studies as as evidence of a food allergy "epidemic".

5 Anon, "Better information urgently needed as childhood peanut allergy rate climbs," *ASCIA* (Feb. 25, 2009). http://www.allergy.org.au/content/view/360/76/

6 R.J. Mullins, "Characteristics of childhood peanut allergy in the Australian Capital Territory 1995 to 2007," *J Allergy and Clin Immunol.*, 123, 3 (March, 2009): 689-693.

7 Linda Smith, Op. cit.

8 Linda Smith, Op. cit.

9 A. Kemp, "Severe peanut allergy in Australian children," *Med J of Australia,* 183, 5 (2005): 277; A.L. Ponsonby, et al., "A prospective study of the association between home gas appliance use during infancy and subsequent dust mite sensitization and lung function in childhood," *Clin Exp Allergy*, 31 (2001): 1544-1552.

10 A team from McGill University conducted the first temporal survey of peanut allergy in North America. In 2000/2002, they surveyed 4,339 schoolchildren in Montreal and found that 1.5% percent of the children in kindergarten through third grade - between the ages of 5 and 9 - had peanut and/or nut allergies. In a 5-year follow-up study they found that prevalence of this allergy had increased to 1.71% in 2005/07. In 5 years prevalence of peanut allergy in Montreal children had increased 35%. This may hold true for all Canadian children. A survey of anaphylaxis in 2000-01 in Canada indicated that 1.44% of the pediatric population under 17 years had portable, Epipen epinephrine dispensed. This was believed to under-represent teens and reflect an underestimation of true occurrence rate of anaphylaxis. F. Estelle, et al., "Allergy Frontiers and Futures," *Allergy Clin Immunol Int.,* 242, 1 (2004).

11 M. Ben-Shoshan, et al., "Is the prevalence of peanut allergy increasing? A five-year follow-up study on the prevalence of peanut allergy in Montreal school children aged 5 to 9 years," *The Journal of Allergy and Clinical Immunology*, 121, 2, (Feb., 2008): S97.

12 N.E. Eriksson, et al., "Self-reported food hypersensitivity in Sweden, Denmark, Estonia, Lithuania and Russia," *J Invest Allergol Clin Immunol.*, 14 (2004): 70-79.

13 In France, a 2002 study of children in Toulouse schools found that 6.7% of all children had true food allergies, this compared to the 4.7% of US children. Cow milk, eggs and peanuts were the main foods reported where 8.2% of children of all ages reported having an adverse reaction to peanut. It was unclear as to the exact percentage anaphylactic to peanut. Overall, the rate of peanut sensitization could be between 1.05% and 2.5% of the overall population. 18% of the population of France was under 15 in 2002 indicating that .45% of children were allergic to peanuts. F. Rancé, "Prevalence and main characteristics of schoolchildren diagnosed with food allergies in France," *Clinical and Experimental Allergy*, 35, 2 (Feb., 2005): 167-172.

14 M. Morisset, et al., "Prevalence of peanut sensitization in a population of 4,137 patients referred to allergologists," *AllergoVigilance Network* (2002). http://www.cicbaa.com/pages_us/allergovigilance/prevalencepeanut.pdf

15 A. Mehl, et al., "Anaphylactic reactions in children – a questionnaire-based survey in Germany," *Allergy*, 60, 11 (Nov., 2005):1440-1445.

16 C. Roehr, et al., "Food allergy and non-allergic food hypersensitivity in children and adolescents," *Clin Exp Allergy*, 34, 1 (Oct., 2004): 1534-41.

17 T.F. Leung, et al., "Parent-reported adverse food reactions in Hong Kong Chinese pre-schoolers: epidemiology, clinical spectrum and risk factors," *Pediatric Allergy & Immunology*, 20, 4 (June, 2009): 339-346. About 3800 children ages 2-7 living in Hong Kong were recruited. Parents reported 8.1%

adverse food reactions and doctors confirmed 4.6%. Top 3 causes of AFR were shellfish, egg, peanut (8.1%). AFR is a common atopic disorder in Hong Kong pre-school children, and prevalence rates are comparable to Caucasians. Mainland China fewer parent reported AFR in 4%.

18 R. Hatahet, et al., "Sensibilisation aux allergens d'arachide chez les nourrissons de moins de quarter mois: à propos de 125 observations," *Rev Fr Allergol Immunol Clin.*, 34 (1994): 377-81.

19 D.J. Hill, et al., "Clinical spectrum of food allergy in children in Australia and South-East Asia: identification and targets for treatment," *Annals of Medicine*, 31, 4 (Aug., 1999): 272-81. Despite the high rate of peanut consumption it is a are allergen. Allergy to all foods affects 3.4% to 5% of the residents in Beijing, Guangdong, and the Sheng-Li oil fields. Top allergens include fish, shrimp, crab and seaweed. In 29 children aged two to 12 years with diagnosed food allergy in the Chinese population studied, none had signs of clinical allergy to peanut, although 2% of them were skin-test positive to peanut in 1999.

20 T.F. Leung, "Sensitization to common food allergens is a risk factor for asthma in young Chinese children in Hong Kong," *Journal of Asthma*, 39, 6 (Sept. 2002): 523-9.

21 K., Beyer K, et al., "Effects of cooking methods on peanut allergenicity," *J Allergy Clin Immunol.*, 107, 6 (2001): 1077-1081.

22 Mangala M. Pai, Assist. Prof., Centre for Basic Sciences, KMC, Mangalore, Bejai "Peanut allergy – prevention?" *BMJ* (Sept., 2006).

23 D. Aaronov, et al., "Natural history of food allergy in infants and children in Israel," *Ann Allergy Asthma Immunol.*, 101, 6 (Dec., 2008): 637-40.

24 G. Du Toit, Op. cit.

25 D. Aaronov, Op. cit.

26 M. Ebisawa, et al., "Food allergy in Japan," *Allergy Clin Immunol Int.*,15 (May, 2003): 214-7.

27 C.G Mortz, et al., "The prevalence of peanut sensitisation and the association to pollen sensitization in a cohort of unselected adolescents," *Pediatric Allergy & Immunology*, 16, 6 (Sept., 2005):501-506.

28 Ibid.

29 C. Crooks, et al., "The changing epidemiology of food allergy, implications for New Zealand," *The New Zealand Medical Journal*, 121, 1271 (April 4, 2008)

30 D.J. Hill, et al., "The frequency of food allergy in Australia and Asia," *Environmental Toxicology and Pharmacology*, 4, 1-2 (Nov., 1997): 101-110.

31 L. Shek Pei-Chi, Op. cit. http://www.med.nus.edu.sg/paed/academic/AP_food_allergy.htm

32 C. Crooks, et al., Op. cit.

33 Sweden exhibits a very high prevalence of peanut allergy but Denmark and Norway very low. Per capita consumption of peanut in Sweden is low at .8kg per person compared with 2.1kg in the US. In a study of children who were tested for IgE antibodies for peanut between Jan. 1994 and 1998, authors found similar course of events for young children under 6 in the US. Occurrence of peanut allergy had increased without a country wide increase in consumption. J. Van Odijk, et al., "Specific immunoglobulin E antibodies to peanut over time in relation to peanut intake, symptoms and age," *Pediatric Allergy & Immunolog,*15, 5 (Oct., 2004): 442-448.

34 J. Van Odijk, et al., "Specific IgE antibodies to peanut in western Sweden; has the occurrence of peanut allergy increased without an increase in consumption?" *Allergy*, 56, 6 (June, 2001): 573-7.

35 British Society for Allergy & Clinical Immunology http://www.bsaci.org

36 The UK has shown the highest prevalence of peanut allergy in the world. The LEAP has stated that 1 in 70 UK children suffers from peanut allergy and that the vast majority (80%) will have the allergy for life. In a population based study of 3 year olds in the UK, the prevalence of sensitization to peanuts increased from 1.3 percent to 3.2 percent between 1989 and1995. In 1998, the UK Dept. of Health recommended that mothers from "high risk" families (those with a history of atopy) avoid eating peanuts during pregnancy and lactation and that they not give their infants peanut products for the first three years of life. Isle of Wight study at the David Hide Asthma and Allergy Research Centre found that the numbers of children who tested positive for peanut tripled between 1989 and 1996: 1.1% of children in 1989 compared to 3.3% in 1996. J. Grundy, et al. "Rising prevalence of allergy to peanut in children: data from 2 sequential cohorts," *J Allergy Clin Immunol*, 110 (2002): 784-9.

37 J. Grundy, et al., "Peanut allergy in three year old children – a population based study," *J. Allergy Clin Immunol.*, 107 (2001): S231.

38 Committee on Toxicity of Chemicals in Food, Consumer Products, and the Environment, *Peanut allergy* (London: Department of Health, 1998) 1-57.

39 Prevalence of peanut and tree nut allergy in US was determined by a telephone survey with a 5 year follow up. A team of researchers found that the rate of peanut/tree nut allergies increased significantly in children but not at all in adults. The number of allergic children had doubled from .6% in 1997 to 1.2% in 2002. And one of the most puzzling facts is that 9% of Americans had "serologic evidence" of sensitivity to peanuts according to the CDC's National Health and Nutrition Examination Survey (NHANE III data was collected from 1988 to 1994). S.H. Sicherer, et al. "Prevalence of peanut and tree nut allergy in the United States determined by means of a random digit dial telephone survey: a 5-year follow up study," *The Journal of Allergy and Clinical Immunology*," 112, 6 (Dec. 2003,): 1203-1207; S. Sicherer, et al., "Prevalence of peanut and tree nut allergy in the US determined by a random digit dial telephone survey," *J of Allergy and Clin Immunology*, 103 (1999): 559-62.

40 A.M. Barnum, S.L. Lukacs, "Food allergy among U.S. children: trends in prevalence and hospitalizations," National Center for Health Statistics, CDC (Oct. 22, 2008). In 2003, 4.7% of children less than five years had food allergies and about 6% to 8 % of children younger than 4. Since 1998, there had been an 18% increase.

41 DeNoon, DJ. "Food allergy in kids up 18%," *MedicineNet.com* (Oct. 22, 2008).

42 Mike Stobbe, "Food allergies increasing in US kids," *SF Gate* (Oct. 22, 2008). The CDC used data from a National Health Interview Survey which sampled 9,500 children in 2007 and the National Hospital Discharge Survey which includes 270,000 inpatient records from 500 hospitals.

43 L. Chiu L, "Estimation of the sensitization rate to peanut by prick skin test in the general population: results from the National Health and Nutrition Examination Survey, 1980-1994," *J Allergy Clin Immunol.*, 107 (2001): S192.

44 S. Sicherer, S., et al. "Prevalence of Peanut and Tree Nut Allergy in the US determined by a Random Digit Dial Telephone Survey," Op. cit.

Index

in vaccines, 8, 61, 114, 121-128, 142-145

and the World Health Organisation, 26, 60, 115-116, , 124-125, 145

Peanut allergy

acceleration, 6, 17-18, 21, 28, 55-56, 73, 129-138, 146-148, 159

age of onset 40-41

arrival, 13, 21, 64, 112-115, 120, 128, 151-152

and atopy, 36-38

and breast feeding, 32-36

bully, 25

deaths, 13, 14-19, 123, 126, 128, 146

and the gastro-intestinal tract, 5, 7, 35-36, 52, 63-64, 97

and gender 28, 42-43, 50, 55

and genetics 49-50, 60, 153-154

and geography, 28-36, 63-64

and heredity, 2, 49-52,

hysteria, 25

and the legal system 24-25

and maternal diet, 4, 32-36

media, 12-18, 126, 128

and mice, 50, 58, 65, 148-149

person most at risk for, 28, 152-155

resolution, 54-55

and race, 43-44

statistics, 1, 17-19, 29-31, 54-55, 138, 150-152, 167-171

in schools, 1, 20-23

and Th1-Th2 Paradigm, 38-40, 49, 52-54, 61, 67, 73-74

and toxicity, 28, 56, 64-68, 126, 148-150, 152-154

treatments, 19-20

and vaccination, 6-8, 37-38, 51-52, 79, 121-129, 138-139, 141-154, 164

Penicillin

allergy, 113-117

history, 14, 112-117

and peanut oil, 113-117, 120, 155

Pharmaceutical industry

history, 14-16, 87-95

nostrum remedium, 89, 91

sales & marketing, 89-91, 127, 163

profitability, 9, 21, 25-26, 90-91, 93-95, 136, 163

consumers, 26, 60, 90-95, 142-146

use of peanut oil, 26, 57-61, 113-128, 155

and law, 26, 87, 127, 144-146, 152, 159-160

Profet, Margie, 7, 64-68, 70, 75, 148, 152

R

Richet, Charles, 7, 80, 102-105, 157

Romansky, Monroe J., 114-117, 120, 122, 125, 128, 155

Russia, 30, 63, 83, 87, 151, 168

S

Sabrina's Law, 24

Serum sickness, 79, 92, 97-102, 108, 115, 129, 148, 155

Shaw, George Bernard, 101-102, 164

Singapore, 29-31, 44, 63, 146, 150, 170

Social Problem, The, 81

Sweden, 4, 30, 32, 83, 155, 171

T

Th1-Th2 Paradigm, 38-40, 49, 52-54, 61, 67, 73-74

Technological innovation, 80-81, 84-86

Thimerosal, 143, 159-162

Toxin Hypothesis, 7, 56, 64-68, 70-71

U

UK, 8, 17-19, 25, 28-30, 33-36, 44-45, 48, 63, 87, 126, 129, 137-138, 152, 170

and Adjuvant 65, 126

Isle of Wight, 18

Unvaccinated, 52-53, 142, 157

US 88-95, 97-99, 110-118, 129-132, 135-136, 151-153, 155-158

peanut allergy statistics, 1, 4, 29, 166

ER records 17, 138

FDA, 13-14, 59-60, 125-126, 133, 135, 142, 145

Vaccination rates, 8, 52-53